EBOLA VIRUS
and WEST AFRICA

The EBOLA VIRUS and WEST AFRICA

Medical and Sociocultural Aspects

Dr. Felix I. Ikuomola

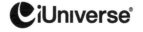

THE EBOLA VIRUS AND WEST AFRICA
MEDICAL AND SOCIOCULTURAL ASPECTS

Copyright © 2015 Dr. Felix I. Ikuomola.

All rights reserved. No part of this book may be used or reproduced by any means, graphic, electronic, or mechanical, including photocopying, recording, taping or by any information storage retrieval system without the written permission of the publisher except in the case of brief quotations embodied in critical articles and reviews.

iUniverse books may be ordered through booksellers or by contacting:

iUniverse
1663 Liberty Drive
Bloomington, IN 47403
www.iuniverse.com
1-800-Authors (1-800-288-4677)

Because of the dynamic nature of the Internet, any web addresses or links contained in this book may have changed since publication and may no longer be valid. The views expressed in this work are solely those of the author and do not necessarily reflect the views of the publisher, and the publisher hereby disclaims any responsibility for them.

Any people depicted in stock imagery provided by Thinkstock are models, and such images are being used for illustrative purposes only.
Certain stock imagery © Thinkstock.

ISBN: 978-1-4917-7130-3 (sc)
ISBN: 978-1-4917-7131-0 (e)

Library of Congress Control Number: 2015910737

Print information available on the last page.

iUniverse rev. date: 07/10/2015

Dedication

This Ebola Virus and West Africa book is dedicated to Ebola survivors, those that fought against Ebola, and all Ebola-related deaths and most especially Dr. John Taban Dada, one of my best friends and colleagues at John F. Kennedy Medical Center, Monrovia, Liberia that contracted Ebola while providing care for patients with Ebola and subsequently died on October 9, 2014 due to Ebola Virus Disease (EVD) in Liberia.

Though Ebola had done its worst by snatching innocent souls away, we will do our best through this book to make good your ultimate sacrifices and to be your voice to say, "Never again to Ebola outbreaks in West Africa."

Contents

Dedication v
List of Illustrations xv
List of Tables xvii
Foreword xix
Preface xxi
Acknowledgements xxiii
Introduction xxv

Chapter One: Ebola in Brief 1
What is Ebola? 1
   Definition 1
   Incubation period 1
Ebola Historical account 1
Ebola in West Africa 3

Chapter Two: Background Information 5
Ebola Epidemiology 5
   Ebola classification 5
   Other hemorrhagic diseases 5
   Transmission 6
      Animal-Animal 6
      Animal-human 6
      Human-human 7
   Disease burden 7
      Morbidity 7
      Mortality 7
      Fatality rate 8
   Economic burden 8
      Direct 9
      Indirect 9
Pathogenesis 10
   Clinical features 10
   Investigations 10
   Diagnosis 11
   Treatment 11

Differential Diagnosis 12
Complications 12
Prognosis 12

Chapter Three: West Africa: People, Politics, and Policy 13
Geography 13
Cultural practices 14
    Tribes 14
    Traditional practices 15
Labor and trade 16
    Free movement 16
    Family Inter-border settlements 16
    High level of unemployment 17
Education 17
Religion 18
History of Social conflicts and wars 19
Lack of trust between the governed and the governors 19
    Lack of transparency 19
    Bribery and corruption 20
    Lack of accountability 20
    Failed political promises 20
    Tax evasion 21
    Repressive policy
    Nepotism 21

Chapter Four: West African Pre-Ebola Status 22
Health infrastructures 22
    Physician-Patient ratio 22
    Malfunctioning Health facilities
    Insufficient health centers 23
    Lack of health insurance 23
    Low GDP on health 23
    Traditional medicinal practitioners 24
Nutrition 24
    Unbalanced diet 24
    Bat-eaters 25
    Bush-meat eaters 25
    Compromised immunity 25
Poor Road infrastructures 25

Poor Social amenities 26
    Water.. 26
    Communication 27
    Lack of social security system 28

Chapter Five: West African Intra-Ebola Situation............................ 29
Poor preparation.. 29
    Lack of promptly designated isolation centers 29
    Deficient infectious disease training....................................... 29
Lack of resources 29
    Lack of personal protective equipment (PPE) 29
    Insufficient fund 30
Politico-security instability 30
Conflicting Ebola message 30
False traditional health attendant claims 31
Lack of faith in Government health message 33
Ebola-spread-enhancing cultural practices... 33
    Burial ritual 33
        Corpse-washing... 33
        Preservation of certain parts 34
        Holding and wailing on the corpse 34
    Lack of hygiene 34
    Eating customs 35
    Sharing sleeping bed with the sick....................................... 35
    Greeting norms... 36
        Hugging... 36
        Kissing 36
    Living Conditions... 36
        Family living together.. 36
        Overcrowding.. 37
    Magnanimous norms 37
        Bush meat sharing 37
        Other food stuff sharing 37
    Anti-sociocultural consideration of Ebola isolation 37
    Cultural importance of burial ground or cemetery................ 38
        Social unacceptability of cremation 38
        Social discrimination if family burial site is unknown
        or if the burial rite is undone 39

Bat	39
Food	39
Traditional medicinal importance	40
Traditional religion	40
Sharing of deceased personal belongings	41
Stealing of Ebola isolation materials	41
Power of money and Position	41
Ebola fraud	42
Ebola Diagnostic Difficulty	42
Mimic other diseases	42
Wrong diagnosis	42
Lack of well-equipped laboratory	42
Lengthy days before diagnostic results	42
Other diseases' negligence	43
Travel restrictions, quarantine	43
School closure	43
Ebola screening	44
Port of entry and exit	44
Local unscientific preventive measures	44
High salt solution ingestion	44
High Bitter kola nut consumption	45
Media role	46
Assistance	47
United Nations (UN)	47
United States of America (USA)	47
United Kingdom (UK)	48
France	48
Economic Community of West Africa States (ECOWAS)	48
African Union (AU)	49
World Bank	49
Non-Governmental Organization (NGO)	49
Chapter Six: West African Post-Ebola State	**51**
Depletion of the meagre health resources	51
Lower GDP on health	51
Reduced Physician-Patient ratio	51
Orphans	52
Reduced orthodox health patronage	52
More traditional health attendant patronage	53

Reduced economy 53
   Reduced workforce 54
   Working hour loss 54
      Sickness 54
      Quarantine 54
      Isolation 55
      Disability 55
Ebola myth 55
Social Stigmatization 56
Post-Ebola syndrome 56
Possible short-lived Ebola surveillance 57
Ebola-free declaration's milestone 57
   Senegal 57
   Nigeria 59
   Mali 61
Possible vaccine 62
Possible therapeutics 63
Possible Mutations 66

Chapter Seven: Ebola multifactorial prognostic measures 67
Ebola pattern of transmission and outbreak-type-prognostic factors 67
General Ebola Eradication Prognostic factor 68

**Chapter Eight: Ethical issues in using unregistered
        interventions for EVD** 70
Ethical Dilemmas in Ebola outbreaks 70
Ethics and Interventions 70
   Historical accounts of ethics in research 70
   Fundamental ethical principles 71
Argument for ethical issues in using unregistered interventions
for EVD in West Africa 72
   Ethical rationale argument 72
   Relevant facts 73
   Resolution effects 74
   Relevant ethical considerations 75
Argument against ethical issues in using unregistered interventions
for EVD in West Africa 78
   Ethical disagreement 78
   Interventions' efficacy unpredictability 79

  Possible severe adverse events...80
  Ethical soundness versus ethical acceptability 80
Discussion..81
  Application of Ethics...81
  Scientific integrity 82
  Pragmatism..83
  Double set-up..84
Bioethical Summary..84
  Balancing ethics, science, and pragmatism 84
  Balancing Hippocratic Oath and reciprocity and social usefulness.....85
  Professional obligations..85

Chapter Nine: Prevention and Control of Ebola 86
Public guidelines 86
Health workers/ Care givers guidelines...86
Laboratory Guidelines...87
Animal guidelines 87
Travel warnings..87

Chapter Ten: Ebola-related Memories..88
Storylines 88
Health-care delivery system in Africa 100

Chapter Eleven: New West Africa: Preventing
  Ebola Historical Repetition...106
Cultural evolution, revolution, and resolution 106
Traditional healer incorporation Program 118
Integration of African traditional health into Medical curriculum 118
Professional responsibility in fighting Ebola outbreaks 119
West African Health Organization (WAHO).....................................121
Outbreak responder training..122
Basic amenities and infrastructure improvement 123
Decentralization...124
Rapid Ebola test kits 124
Training courses, workshops, and simulation exercises 125
Border Health facilities...125
Basic Approach to getting things done successfully in Africa............126

Chapter Twelve: Conclusion 131
Hippocratic Oath 131
Medico-Cultural disease 131
Never Again 131

List of Abbreviations 135
Bibliography 137
List of Contributors 177
Index 179
Epilogue 185

List of Illustrations

Figure 1: West Africa and Ebola Virus Disease
Figure 2: Ebola Origin
Figure 3: Fruit bat Taxonomy
Figure 4: Ebola Transmission
Figure 5: Schematic Diagram of Ebola Virus
Figure 6: Schematic Map of West Africa
Figure 7: Ifa Divination
Figure 8: African Traditional Chief
Figure 9: Trade in Africa
Figure 10: African Incantation
Figure 11: Effect of War and Social Conflict
Figure 12: Radio Health Talk in Sierra Leone
Figure 13: A temporary Shelter
Figure 14: Table Salt
Figure 15: Bitter Kola nut
Figure 16: Dr. David Koroma
Figure 17: Trinida Kollie-Jones
Figure 18: Dr. Felix Ikuomola
Figure 19: Wendy Ikuomola
Figure 20: Dr. Olumide Oluwarotimi
Figure 21: Internet Use in Africa
Figure 22: Road to Forest in Africa
Figure 23: Man at work in Africa
Figure 24: Ancient communicating drum in Africa
Figure 25: Mobile Phone user in Africa
Figure 26: Chewing stick use in Africa
Figure 27: Toothbrush and toothpaste use in Africa
Figure 28: Speedboat use in Africa
Figure 29: Canoes in Africa
Figure 30: Local fishing net
Figure 31: Community engagement
Figure 32: Professional responsibility
Figure 33: Modern Laboratory Equipment
Figure 34: Well Equipped Laboratory

List of Tables

1. Ebola Timeline
2. Comparative Ebola Distribution
3. Ebola Laboratory Panels
4. West Africa and Water and Sanitation
5. West African Countries and Communications
6. March 25, 2014-March 29, 2015 Ebola Distribution
7. Ebola and Health workers in West Africa
8. Potential Ebola Vaccines - VSV - EBOV
9. Possible drugs for patients with EVD
10. Ebola pattern of transmission and outbreak-type-prognostic factors
11. General Ebola Eradication Prognostic factor
12. Socio-Cultural Evolution, Revolution, and Resolution

Foreword

We have failed in properly managing Ebola in Africa. This excellent review discusses cultural issues not reflected in the current literature. Dr Ikuomola, a well-educated African physician, provides us with perceptions and facts that can significantly impact outcome. He also addresses what must be done to succeed in our quest to successfully treat this challenging problem. Culture must be considered in all our management programs. Frequently it is not even considered - or what is proposed is incorrect. Dr Ikuomola expertly provides us with a cultural foundation that currently remains unreported and unintegrated to our knowledge.

Professor Rosanne Harrigan
Chair, Dept. of Complementary and Alternative Medicine
Director, Faculty Development Program,
Director, Clinical Research Program,
John A. Burns School of Medicine,
University of Hawaii at Manoa,
Honolulu, HI, USA.

Preface

It has always been true that little attention has been given to the undeniable impact of socio-cultural factors on communicable disease. In fact, most of the preparatory and intensive training of health personnel attending to the needs of those societies where culture is at the center of life have given only lip service to the importance of integrating this culture into the medical training curriculum. I was born in a culturally saturated community, attended an advanced school in a culture-oriented city, and obtained my medical degree from a university whose motto is "for learning and culture." Having worked in and traveled to many countries enabled me to further confirm the significance of cultural in the medical world. This book, *Ebola Virus and West Africa, Medical and Sociocultural aspects,* fills in the deficiency of cultural information, innovation, and integration. Culture plays a major role in the large-scale spread of Ebola outbreaks in West Africa and it is also indispensable to Ebola containment, surveillance, prevention, and screening.

Felix Ikuomola

Acknowledgements

I am very grateful to God Almighty for His providence. I am thankful to Dr Beatriz Rodriguez who first asked me to do a PowerPoint presentation on Ebola in 2014 and asked me to write an article on Ebola in 2015. After submitting the outlines to her, she came back to inform me that Dr Rosanne Harrigan said that the outlines would be good for a book, hence the birth of this book on Ebola, a medico-cultural disease. Special thanks to Dr Rosanne Harrigan for her leadership and guidance and Dr Deborah Kissinger who motivated me to add the bioethics section. Special heart-felt thankfulness to my wife, Wendy Ikuomola, who always encourages me even when I engage in a herculean task such as the writing of this sociocultural impact of Ebola outbreaks in West Africa. I am also very thankful to my mother, who has always been so supportive and caring since the death of my father when I was just seven years old. Special thanks to CDC, WHO, UN, ECOWAS, MSF, and other authors whose tremendous works have contributed greatly to the success story of this Ebola Virus and West Africa book.

I am also very grateful to Dr Walter Thompson for his initial review, advice, and final editing of the book, Dr David Koroma for immense contributions on Ebola outbreak in Sierra Leone, Trinida Kollie-Jones for her wonderful and personal story on how she lost her childhood friends and others to Ebola in Liberia, Dr Olumide Oluwarotimi for perspectives of Ebola in Nigeria, and Chief Oyetade Akintubuwa (Olukoyi), the head of the Alaghoro of Ugbo Kingdom, a renowned historian who contributed greatly to the African traditional practice aspect. Special thanks to Dr Beatriz Rodriguez, Dr Rosanne Harrigan, Natalie Zwing, Marshal Akintubuwa, Otunba Gbenga Ikuomola, and my family for their support for the publication of the book. Special gratitude to Dr Jerris Hedges, the Dean of John A. Burns School of Medicine (JABSOM) of University of Hawaii and Acting Director of University of Hawaii Cancer Center, Honolulu, Hawaii, USA for his professional review and vital comments. Finally to all that will be reading this book, I acknowledge your flair for a medico-cultural book.

Introduction

Ebola had never been heard of in West Africa before. We in West Africa always thought it was a disease of East Africa. But this assumption failed to hold on March 25, 2014 when the World Health Organization (WHO) alerted the whole world that there was an Ebola outbreak in Guinea. It was like a bad dream to many of us in West Africa! The question on every lip was, "Is it true?" We were all caught unaware. How did Ebola find itself on the beautiful shores of West Africa? Why did it decide to leave the East coast of Africa and head to the West coast? Believe you me, we were not prepared! It was the least expected among the diseases we ever heard of. We were used to malaria fever, typhoid fever, meningitis, diarrhea, and malnutrition, not Ebola. Before it fully dawned on us that Ebola was real, it had claimed not only lives of innocent citizens of West Africa, but our health practitioners as well.

Our traditional African healers thought traditional medicines and incantations would confront the power of Ebola, before they knew, Ebola had started claiming their lives as well.

This book is intended to enlighten us about Ebola, African culture, and medicine. It further opens our minds to the state of the health infrastructure; African tradition before Ebola struck; the role sociocultural factors played in spreading Ebola; the role they played in containment, and the need to integrate traditional African medicinal practice into modern medicine and collaborate together for the betterment of the society.

The book will also arouse your curiosity to the importance of culture in disease transmission, treatment, prevention, and control. It will serve as a stepping stone for your quest for exploration of medico-cultural disease worldwide, and why some people do things the way they are culturally tailored.

This book has a section that is devoted to Ebola-related personal stories and some works that had been done in other parts of Africa. The contributors to this section presented touchy and emotional accounts of Ebola in Liberia, Sierra Leone, and Nigeria.

Chapter One
Ebola in Brief

What is Ebola?

Definition: Ebola is a virus that belongs to the family Filoviridae and genus Ebolavirus. Ebola Virus Disease (EVD), formerly known as Ebola hemorrhagic fever, can often cause an acute, fatal life-threatening condition.[1,2]

Incubation period: From the time of the infection with the virus to the onset of the disease symptom takes 2 to 21 days.[2]

Ebola Historical account

Nzara, Sudan and Yambuku, Democratic Republic of Congo (DRC, formerly Zaire) had simultaneous Ebola outbreaks in 1976.[3] The Ebola virus was discovered by Peter Piot, a Belgian scientist.[3,4] Ebola got its name from the Ebola River that is close to Yambuku, DRC.[3,4] Between September 1 and October 24, 1976, 318 unconfirmed and confirmed cases of Ebola hemorrhagic fever occurred in Congo of which 280 died with fatality rate of 88%[1,3] (See Table 1).

Table 1: Ebola Timeline[1]

When	Where	What	Morbidity	Mortality	Fatality
Aug.-Nov. 2014	DR Congo	Zaire virus	66	47	74%
Mar. 2014-Mar. 2015	W. Africa, EU, US	Zaire virus	25213	10460	41.5%
Nov. 2012-Jan. 2013	Uganda	Sudan virus	6*	3*	50%
Jun.-Nov. 2012	DR Congo	Bundibugyo v.	36*	13*	36.1%

Jun.-Oct. 2012	Uganda	Sudan virus	11*	4*	36.4%
May 2012	Uganda	Sudan virus	1	1	100%
Dec. 2008-Feb. 2009	DR Congo	Ebola virus	32	15	47%
Nov. 2008	Philippines	Reston virus	6	0	0%
Dec. 2007-Jan. 2008	Uganda	Bundibugyo v.	149	37	25%
2007	DR Congo	Ebola virus	264	187	71%
2004	Russia	Ebola virus	1	1	100%
2004	Sudan (S. Sudan)	Sudan virus	17	7	41%
Nov.-Dec. 2003	Rep. of Congo	Ebola virus	35	29	83%
Dec. 2002-Apr. 2003	Rep. of Congo	Ebola virus	143	128	89%
Oct. 2001-Mar. 2002	Rep. of Congo	Ebola virus	57	43	75%
Oct. 2001-Mar. 2002	Gabon	Ebola virus	65	53	82%
2000-2001	Uganda	Sudan virus	425	224	53%
1996	Russia	Ebola virus	1	1	100%
1996	Philippines	Reston virus	0	0	0
1996	USA	Reston virus	0	0	0
1996	South Africa	Ebola virus	2	1	50%
Jan. 1996-Jul. 1997	Gabon	Ebola virus	60	45	74%
Jan-Apr. 1996	Gabon	Ebola virus	37	21	57%
1995	DR Congo (Zaire)	Ebola virus	315	250	81%

1994	Côte d'Ivoire (I.C.)	Taï Forest virus	1	0	0%
1994	Gabon	Ebola virus	52	31	60%
1992	Italy	Reston virus	0	0	0
1989-1990	Philippines	Reston virus	3	0	0
1990	USA	Reston virus	4	0	0
1989	USA	Reston virus	0	0	0
1979	Sudan (S. Sudan)	Sudan virus	34	22	65%
1977	Zaire	Ebola virus	1	1	100%
1976	England	Sudan virus	1	0	0%
1976	Sudan (South Sudan)	Sudan virus	284	151	53%
1976	Zaire (DR Congo)	Ebola virus	318	280	88%

*Numbers reflect laboratory confirmed cases only.[1]

Ebola in West Africa

On March 25, 2014, the WHO announced that Ministry of Health in Guinea had reported EVD outbreak of 86 suspected cases that included 59 deaths.[2] The index EVD case was believed by researchers to have started in Meliandou village in Guéckédou Prefecture, Guinea in December 2013.[5] EVD spread more rapidly in West Africa than when it was first noticed in East Africa.[2] See Figure 1.

Fig. 1: West Africa and Ebola Virus Disease

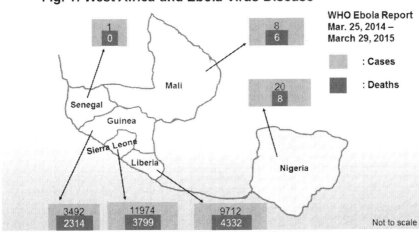

Chapter Two
Background Information

Ebola Epidemiology

Ebola classification: The EVD belongs to the virus family called Filoviridae with three genera which are Cuevavirus, Marburgvirus, and Ebolavirus.[2] In the genus Ebolavirus there are five identified species that include Zaire, Bundibugyo, Sudan, Reston and Taï Forest[2] (See Fig. 2). The first three, Zaire virus, Bundibugyo ebolavirus, and Sudan ebolavirus have been implicated in large Ebola outbreaks in Africa while the last two, Reston and Tai Forest are not known to cause epidemic.[2,6] The 2014 West African Ebola outbreak is known to be caused by Zaire virus species.[2]

Fig. 2: Ebola Origin

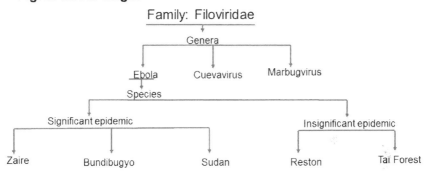

Other hemorrhagic diseases: Viral hemorrhagic fevers (VHFs) is a severe multisystem syndrome affecting multiple body organ systems that is characterized by damage to the body's overall vascular system and impairment of the body's regulatory ability.[6] The term VHF is used to apply to disease caused by Arenaviridae (Lassa fever, Junin and Machupo), Bunyaviridae (Crimean-Congo haemorrhagic fever, Rift Valley Fever, Hantaan haemorrhagic fevers), and Flaviviridae (yellow fever, dengue, Omsk haemorrhagic fever, Kyasanur forest disease).[7] The hemorrhagic fever viruses are RNA viruses that are covered or enveloped in a fatty (lipid) coating. They are dependent upon insect or animal natural reservoirs for survival.[6]

Transmission

Animal-Animal: Fruit bats which belong to Chordata Phylum, Chiroptera order, Megachiroptera suborder, Pteropodidae family, and Pteropus genus are natural Ebola virus hosts[2,8] (See Fig. 3). Fruit bats that are also called flying foxes do not echolocate so they feed on fruit and nectar. They do not usually pitch in the caves, but roost in trees, a feature that might easily enhance infected fruit bats coming in contact with other animals and humans[8,9] (See Fig. 4). Other animal to animal transmissions have been seen in apes, and monkeys as well[1].

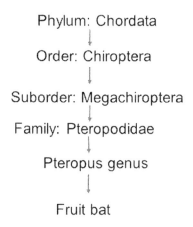

Fig. 3: Fruit bat Taxonomy

Phylum: Chordata
↓
Order: Chiroptera
↓
Suborder: Megachiroptera
↓
Family: Pteropodidae
↓
Pteropus genus
↓
Fruit bat

Animal-human: Humans can become infected when they come in contact with an infected fruit bat, apes, or monkeys, thus promoting animal-human transmission a process called zoonosis.[1] Hunting wild animals for food is a common practice in Africa. Local people often call it bush meat hunting. In the case of the West African Ebola outbreak which was traced to Guinea in December 2014, the international researchers widely believed that an infected bat bit a toddler.[10] It is important to note that there is no scientific evidence to support Ebola virus transmission through mosquitoes or insects.[1] Could it be that Ebola cannot survive in insect internal milieu? Or could it be due to the fact that there is Ebola virucidal fluid in the mosquitoes and other insects that make it impossible for Ebola to multiple and survive, and thus die off? We need more studies to prove the actual mechanism. If it should be true that there is virucidal fluid in mosquitoes against Ebola, then that might be used as an intervention for EVD.

Human-human: Ebola can spread from human-to-human through direct contact (cut skin or mucous membranes that are exposed to infected blood, secretions, organs or other bodily fluids including semen and breast milk) and indirect contact (contaminated surfaces and materials).[1] It has been noted that even men that recovered from Ebola can still transmit Ebola via semen within the first 7 weeks post recovery, so it is advised that men either abstain or use barrier protection within this period if engaged in coital activity.[2] Scientists believed that Ebola cannot be spread by food, by water, or through the air.[1]

Fig. 4: Ebola Transmission

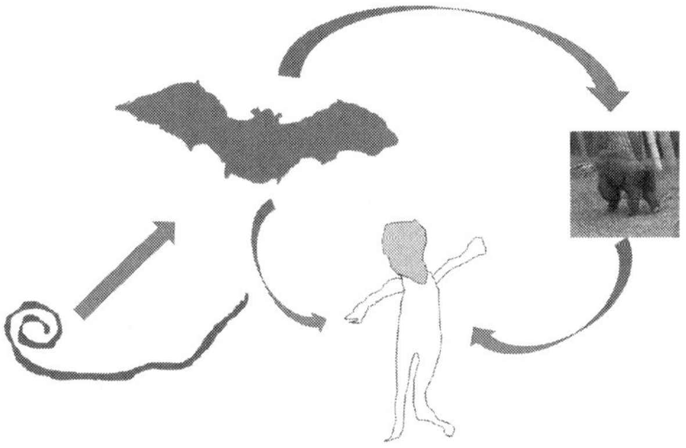

Disease burden

Morbidity: In 1976 when Ebola was first discovered the total cases were 318 over the period of September 1 and November 5.[3] Between 1976 and prior to the West African Ebola outbreaks, the morbidity was 1758 cases,[2] whereas that of the West African Ebola outbreaks that started in March 25, 2014 till March 29, 2015 has infected over 25,213 people[1] (See table 2).

Mortality: The first Ebola virus outbreak in Zaire (Now Democratic Republic of Congo, DRC) in 1976 claimed 280 lives within the period of September 1 and November 5.[3] The deaths recorded between 1976 and prior to the West African Ebola virus outbreak were 1117.[2] However, the death tolls from the West African Ebola that started in March 25, 2014 through March 29, 2015 claimed 10460 which is about 9 times the deaths recorded between 1976 and 2013.[1]

Fatality rate: In 1976, the fatality rate of Ebola virus in Zaire (Congo) was 88% while that of Sudan (Now South Sudan) was 53% and England was 0%.[3] In 1977 the Ebola virus fatality rate seen in Congo was 100%.[3] Currently, the West African Ebola outbreaks have respective fatality rates of 63.5%, 42.5%, 75%, 40%, 0%, and 30.4% in Guinea, Liberia, Mali, Nigeria, Senegal, and Sierra Leone[1] (See table 4). Overall, the fatality rate in West African Ebola outbreaks is about 60%.[1] See tables 2 and 4.

Table 2: Comparative Ebola Distribution		
Outbreaks	Non-West Africa	West Africa
Timeframe	September 1, 1976-March 24, 2014	March 25, 2014-March 29, 2015
Pattern	Intermittently, 38 years	Continuously, 1 year
Strains	Zaire, Sudan, Bundibugyo, Reston, Tai Forest	Zaire
Morbidity	1758	25213
Mortality	1117	10460
Fatality*	25-90%	50%
Comparative Morbidity	1	14.3
Comparative Mortality	1	9.4

* Possibly included unconfirmed cases

Economic burden

Ebola outbreaks in West African sub-regional countries have both direct and indirect economic effects on the public, policy, and politics.[11] The World Bank reported that depending on the extent of the scale and scope of Ebola outbreaks, the two year financial loss impact may range from $3.8 billion (low Ebola) to $32.6 billion (high Ebola) by the end of 2015.[11]

Direct: This includes the cost of government spending on health care, patients' time cost, transportation cost, personal expenses, hospital overhead costs, medical and nursing costs, material and equipment costs, and miscellaneous costs in the health service provision.[11, 12] Ebola has a devastating effect on patient and family savings. Since the early symptoms of Ebola are not different from Malaria or typhoid fever, some of the patients may have spent some money in buying over-the-counter drugs from the local pharmacy and drug store.

Indirect: This includes absenteeism, reduced labor productivity due to workers illness, death, or caring for the sick family or friend.[12,13] The indirect cost on the economy also resulted from "aversion behavior" or "Ebola scare syndrome" where business people or companies, for fear of contacting Ebola, closed down their enterprises, and where some countries even instituted travel restrictions to the mostly Ebola-affected nations.[13] There were also disruptions of the transportation system, agriculture sector, manufacturing, and mining since working together or gathering due to tourism could easily enhance contact with infected individuals or materials.[13]

In Sierra Leone, there were a large employment reduction in wage (9,000) and non-farm self-employed (170,000) workers between July and August 2014 due to Ebola fear.[11] According to the World Bank report on the Ebola economic impact in Sierra Leone there were 40% revenue reduction in non-farm businesses and decrease of non-operational non-farm household enterprise from 12 to 4%.[11]

In Liberia, about half of the household heads were out of work in spite of the fact that construction and heath fields created jobs.[11] The governmental, non-governmental, and private enterprises are responsible for hiring workers in Liberia where most jobs are concentrated in urban areas.[11] Since the Ebola menace, only workers in the public sector in Liberia continue to receive wages while their counterparts in the other hiring sectors were not as fortunate.[11] This is a real economic lost to the household heads.[11] Unfortunately, Ebola outbreaks did not only disable and kill, they also resulted in gender-labor and employment disparity and vulnerability; with men to women respective job loss ratio 2 to 3.[11] Ebola in

Liberia also brought with it increase in cost of living, high food insecurity, and reduction in farming harvest team.[11]

In case of Nigeria, occurrence of Ebola led to closure of shops, thus resulted in fewer customers and commercial businesses.[13] It was projected that the Ebola economic impact could cause the tourist industry a 1% drop in the annual GDP.[13] Of course, due to the reported case of Ebola in Senegal several conferences were cancelled and incoming flights or airlines witnessed fewer passengers.[13] In spite of the fact that there was no reported Ebola case in The Gambia, about 65% of its hotel reservations were canceled and it was also forecasted that if the Ebola outbreaks persisted unabated the tourism and hospitality sectors would be drastically affected.[13]

Pathogenesis

Clinical features: Ebola can present with sudden onset of fever, headache, muscle pain, weakness, sore throat, fatigue, diarrhea, vomiting, abdominal (stomach) pain, rash, and unexplained hemorrhage (bleeding or bruising).[1,2] In taking the history of EVD, travel history and ill contact history are very important in order to raise a high level index of suspicion.[14]

Investigations: Laboratory findings in Ebola patients often include reduced white blood cell and platelet counts and elevated liver enzymes.[2] Prior to the onset of symptoms, most especially fever, Ebola virus may not be detected in blood. In some occasions it may take about three days after the symptoms have started before the Ebola virus can reach detectable levels in patient's blood.[1] Below are the various Ebola laboratory panels (Table 3). See Figure 5 for schematic Ebola virus.

Table 3: Ebola Laboratory Panels

Course of Infection	Laboratory Investigations
Within few days of Ebola symptoms onset	Antigen-capture enzyme-linked immunosorbent assay (ELISA) testing
	IgM ELISA
	Polymerase chain reaction (PCR)
	Virus isolation
Later in disease course or after recovery	IgM and IgG antibodies
Retrospectively in deceased patients	Immunohistochemistry testing
	PCR
	Virus isolation

Laboratory panel[1]

Diagnosis: Since Ebola has many differential diagnoses, laboratory confirmation is the gold standard for definitive Ebola diagnosis[1-3] (See Fig. 5). Ebola can be confirmed through antigen-capture detection tests, antibody-capture enzyme-linked immunosorbent assay (ELISA), serum neutralization test, virus isolation by cell culture, reverse transcriptase polymerase chain reaction (RT-PCR) assay, electron microscopy.[1,15]

Fig. 5: Schematic diagram of Ebola Virus

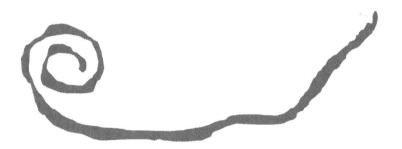

Treatment: Currently, there are no known Ebola-specific therapeutics. What is available for now is only supportive treatment through fluid replacement and symptom-relief measures. However, probable treatments such as blood products, immune therapies, and drug therapeutics are under study and investigation.[1, 15, 16] Likewise, there are no approved vaccines for EVD. However researchers continue to develop vaccines that must pass first through efficacy and human safety testing confirmation.[1, 15]

Differential Diagnosis: Diseases that can present like EVD include malaria, dengue fever, typhoid fever, meningitis, Marburg hemorrhagic fever.[1, 15, 16] Confirmation that symptoms are caused by Ebola virus infection are made using the investigations in Table 3.

Complications: These include shock, coma, joint problems, vision difficulties, multiple organ failure, delirium, and jaundice.[1,17] Other complications may include testicular inflammation, hepatitis, alopecia, fatigue, and neuropathy.[17] Some Ebola survivors may have slow recovery, especially in strength and weight.[17]

Prognosis: Prompt diagnosis, supportive care with fluid replacement, symptom-related treatment and a healthy immune status have been known to contribute to improved chances of survival.[1,15] It has been noticed that individuals that recover from EVD develop antibodies that last for 10 years or more.[1]

Chapter Three
West Africa: People, Politics, and Policy

Geography

The total area covered by West Africa sub-region is about 3.73 million square miles and it is about one-fifth of Africa continent[18]. Africa continent is the second largest continent in the world.[18] West Africa is bordered on the West by the Atlantic Ocean, on the East by Cameroun and Lake Chad, the North by the Sahara, and the South by the Atlantic Ocean.[18] West Africa has a population of about 340 million among 30 major ethnic groups.[18] The fifteen countries that make up West African sub-region include Benin Republic, Burkina Faso, Cape Verde, Cote D'Ivore, Gambia, Ghana, Guinea, Guinea-Bissau, Liberia, Mali, Niger, Nigeria, Senegal, Sierra Leone, and Togo[19] (See Fig. 6). The mission of Economic Community of West Africa States (ECOWAS) was founded in 1975 to "promote economic integration in "all fields of economic activity, particularly industry, transport, telecommunications, energy, agriculture, natural resources, commerce, monetary and financial questions, and social and cultural matters" among the fifteen member states."[19]

Guinea comprises of 24 ethnic groups with a total population of 11.75 million people.[18] Liberia has 16 indigenous tribes and the Americo-Liberia group that only constitutes 5% of the 4.294 million total populations[18]. Sierra Leone consists of 16 ethnic groups with a population of 6.092 million.[18] Guinea, Liberia, and Sierra Leone do not only share borders but also have families that are living across the borders.[18,19]

Fig. 6: Schematic Map of West Africa

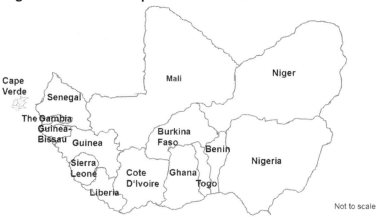

Cultural practices

Tribes: There are about 1000 tribes in West Africa with nearly similar cultural practices.[18, 19] The major ethnic languages in West Africa include but are not limited to Akan, Bassa, Fulani, Hausa, Mende, Yoruba, Ibo, and Zarma.[18, 19]

Fig. 7 Ifa Divination

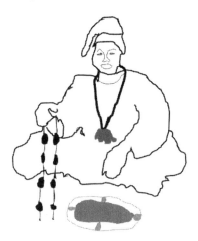

(Ifa divination is a medium of fortune telling or seeking knowlegde of unknown)

Traditional practices: Traditionally, Africans have more respect for the dead than the living.[20,21] As part of African culture, people do not talk bad about the dead no matter how the person might have lived his/her life while on earth.[21] Beginning Immediately after death Africans believe that the dead is higher than the living.[21] Africans also believe that the dead relative is watching over them and they need to take proper care of whatever he/she might have left behind.[20,21] In addition they believe that the dead will bestow special blessings upon them depending on how they regard or treat his/her remains (corpse) and his/her burial site.[21,22] The living will visit the burial site regularly to make sure that the burial site looks nice and neat.[21] At times when a living one has problems which he or she cannot resolve, he/she may decide to go to the burial site to weep or talk at the burial site.[21]

When a very powerful person dies in Africa some cultural practices involve preserving parts of the body of the dead for the next person that will occupy the position left by the deceased.[21] This is usually the practice when a chief, king, or a very significant person dies.[21] The African traditionalists believe that by the preservation of certain parts of the deceased that are handed over through an elaborate ceremony to the next in line to occupy the vacant chieftaincy stool, [21,] the power, influence, knowledge, and wisdom of the deceased powerful person will be transferred to the successor. Some claim that this practice of transfer of power and wisdom from the predecessor to the successor dates back to the time of Elijah in the Bible where Elisha requested a double portion of Elijah's spirit when he was to be taken away from him by the chariots of fire and horses. When the chariots were taking Elijah from him, Elisha got hold of Elijah's garment that got torn into two, and Elisha used the part he had to separate the Jordan River when he was coming back alone (2 Kings 2: 9-14). Body preservation was also practiced by the ancient Egyptians through mummification. [21] Africans also have burial rites which are discussed in other sections.

In some parts of West Africa, female genital mutilation (FGM) is still a practice. Many of the activities associated with this practice appear very attractive.[23] It is also believed by Africans that promote this act that "circumcised" females are less promiscuous. Of course this notion has no proven scientific basis.[23] During the FGM ceremony the same blade is often used for the victims. This practice can easily spread blood-borne diseases.[24]

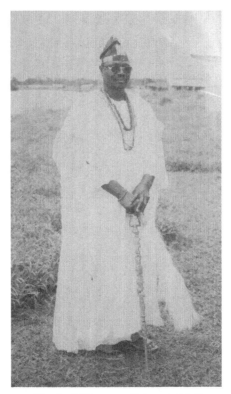

Fig. 8: African traditional chief

Labor and trade

Free movement: The citizens of the member states of ECOWAS have no movement restrictions since they do not require visas to travel from one member state to another.[19]

Accordingly, it is also possible for people to commute from one town to another across borders.

Family Inter-border settlements: There are a lot of inter-border marriages and trade among the neighboring communities that share borders together.[25,26] Even though they may be living in different countries these family members often see themselves as indivisible and inseparable.[26] They do not consider the physical boundaries as barriers[26] but believe that "blood is thicker than water"--a common saying in Africa togetherness.

High level of unemployment: In West Africa the unemployment rate among some member states is as high as 30%; inflation rate is over 11%; and population below poverty line soars over 80%.[18,27] The disconnection between the theory in school and the practical in real life is one of the salient implicating factors in the high level of unemployment in West Africa.[28] The West African development system is not decentralized. It is concentrated in the cities with little job opportunities for those in the villages and rural settlements.[27,28] The available jobs in the West African sub-region cannot support the rate at which the population is exploding, thus the society is witnessing an especially high level of youth unemployment.[27]

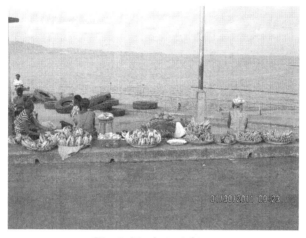

Fig. 9: Trade in Africa

Education

West Africa sub-region has the highest level of illiteracy rates in the world. This hinders economic growth, good governance, health awareness, and prevention of communicable and non-communicable diseases, and reduction of mortality rates. In addition, it interferes with participation in the democratic and governing process according to United Nations Educational, Scientific and Cultural Organization [UNESCO].[29] Literacy is also very important in acquiring the basic knowledge and skills that are needed in order to deal with life challenges, especially in raising children, helping youth, and assisting adults.[29] In most of the West African nations especially in Benin, Burkina Faso, Chad, Ethiopia, Guinea, Mali, Niger, Senegal, Sierra Leone and The Gambia, adult illiteracy is more than 50%.[29]

One of the primary causes of high illiteracy rates in West Africa is ascribed to small amount of GDP that is allocated to education.[29] Many studies have shown strong association between education and health, and that women's education plays a remarkable role in reducing child mortality. The more educated a woman, the less the probability of her child mortality.[30, 31] It is estimated that there is 5-7% child mortality reduction with each corresponding additional year of female schooling.[31, 32]

Religion

Africa, including West Africa, is a very religious society consisting of Christianity, Islam, animism, traditional African religion, and syncretism.[33-35] Traditional African religion is oral-based with no scriptures, reformers, missionaries, or proselytization, but with rituals, magic, shrines, and spiritual activities.[33] Adherents believe in a supreme creator and other gods and goddesses, and in traditional medicine.[33-35] Most African names have meaning and are often related to situations, events, or religion. "*Olusegun*" (Yoruba, Nigeria) means the "Lord is victorious," "*Chukwuemeka*" (Ibo, Nigeria) means "God has done much," and "*Nyamekye*" (Akan, Ghana) means "God's gift."[35] Most Africans in West Africa believe that religion is a way of life and thus religion plays a major role in how they view life and face life challenges including dealing with health and diseases.[33-35]

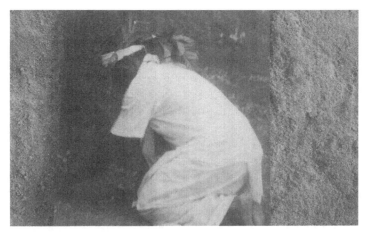

Fig. 10: African Incantation

History of Social conflicts and wars

A few years after Nigeria got her independence from Britain in 1960, a civil war broke out. It lasted for 30 months (1967 to 1970) and claimed over 1 million civilian deaths.[36] Liberia was plunged into civil wars and conflicts for 14 years (1989-1997 and 1999-2003) during which 250,000 lives were lost and 1 million displaced.[28,37] Sierra Leone had civil war for about a decade (1991 to 2002) and the rebels were known for mass rape and mutilations. About 300,000 people were killed and 2.5 million displaced.[28,38] Civil instability due to military coups and counter coups, poor governance, corruption, ethnic marginalization, poverty, and lack of transparency and accountability reduced the pace of development and interfered with the development of a sustainable economic plan and infrastructure in West Africa.[28]

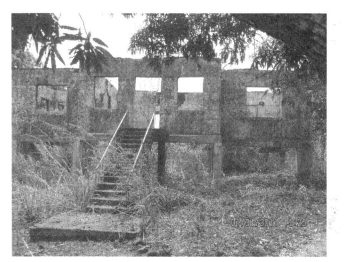

Fig. 11: Effect of war and Social Conflict in Africa

Lack of trust between the governed and the governors

Lack of transparency: As noted by Annan of Kofi Annan International Peacekeeping Training Centre, Ghana wrote in the research article that one of the main problems responsible for civil conflicts and wars in the West Africa sub-region is lack of transparency.[28] Transparency is very vital to building a trusted and last-longing relationship between the governed and the governors.[28] In West Africa transparency is not considered by the leaders, politicians, and policy makers as a necessary ingredient to societal stability and avoidance of conflicts.

Bribery and corruption: These are age-long endemic institutions in West Africa-to the extent that people have come to believe that you cannot get anything done without bribing your way out.[39] Those in public offices expect you to bring them some gifts before you can receive anything from the government, no matter how legitimate the claim you may have. By the same token, those seeking help from the government know that as long as they offer some gifts, whatever they request can be considered done.[40] The appalling and the unfortunate thing about the situation is that children born in West Africa have come to consider bribery and corruption as part of life and one of the norms and values of the society.[39,40] One of the Cote D'Ivoire proverbs, "Mutual gifts cement friendship."[41] There is no doubt, one of the most important parts of African culture is the spirit of giving and appreciation, especially in the agrarian society where visiting farmers bring farm products for the town-dwellers and town-dwellers help the returning farmers with farming tool assistance.[41] Of course, it is different now. Those working in the offices are hired and paid for the jobs they are doing.

Lack of accountability: Generally, West African politicians and leaders consider themselves to be immune to accountability so they do what they want, even engaging in the laundering of the meager resources of the states.[42] The cronies of the leaders also benefit from this ugly culture of impunity.[41, 42] Because there is no entrenched system of accountability in the society, most contracts are awarded to ghost contractors that never carry out any projects.[41-43]

Failed political promises: The electorates are promised heaven and earth during the political electioneering process but immediately after these politicians are elected they turn their backs on those that voted for them.[44] They never engage their constituencies nor report back to the people that elected them into office.[45] The only time they remember the voters is during the election time.[44] Of course, the majority of those in their constituencies are illiterate so it's difficult for them to know what they should be expecting from the politicians or to use the power of their votes to deny any failed political system, party, or individual.[45]

Tax evasion: It is sad to say that West Africa is still deficient of an effective and efficient tax system.[46] Most countries in West Africa practice a flat tax rate where no matter what you earn everyone pays the same amount of tax. This is the usual system that the governments use for unskilled workers.[47] There is no system to enforce it and the only time that the governments ask for the flat tax rate receipt is when the individual has something to do with the public office.[46] There are some countries that are practicing both progressive and flat tax rate systems. It is equally true to say that since the people are not paying taxes to the government, the government has an "I-don't-care-attitude" towards the people as well, probably "law of Karma".

Repressive policy: Most policies in Africa are economic repressive, they are not progressive at all and thus hinder growth and development.[48] In some countries in West Africa, governments have a land use decree or policy that ensures that the land belongs to the governments even though the land is the property of the people.[49,50] Because of this repressive policy even when mineral resources or farming are being done on this land, royalties and the benefits go to the governments directly without proper compensation to the people that originally own the land.[48-51] This contributes in no small measure to the poverty situation in West Africa.

Nepotism: West Africa being a sub-region of tribes also ensures that their tribal people benefit at the expense of competent individuals that do not belong to their tribes.[28] This has been implicated as one of the causes of conflict and wars in the sub-region[28]. Mediocrity breeds sub-optimized output and productivity thereby leading to stunted national growth, impaired technologic advancement, and fragile national stability.[28, 52]

Chapter Four
West African Pre-Ebola Status

Health infrastructures

Physician-Patient ratio: In most countries in West Africa the physician-patient ratio is 1-2 doctors per 100,000 persons with scanty health personnel in the country[18, 53]. As in other parts of the world it takes many years to undergo training to become a doctor.[54] In West Africa the economic doldrums and incessant strikes do not only cause many medical students to spend longer years to qualify but also causes some to drop out for lack of financial support.[28] The stagnant economy in most West African countries affects the wages of medical personnel and thus hinders their ability to update their medical knowledge as well as to acquire advance medical technology and to upgrade obsolete medical tools.[28,55] Another singular factor that contributes to the reduced numbers of doctors in West Africa is brain drain.[55] Currently, Europe and United States have many qualified doctors from West Africa due to foraging for greener pastures.[56] Prior to Ebola outbreaks, Liberia had 4.3 million people with only 51 medical doctors, 978 nurses and midwives, and 269 pharmacists.[57-59] It is believed that Liberia has more Liberian physicians in the US than in Liberia. Sierra Leone has 6 million population with 136 doctors, 1,017 nurses and midwives, and 114 pharmacists, Guinea has 12 million population with 940 physicians, 4408 nurses and midwives, and 190 pharmacists while Nigeria with 170 million population has 58,363 doctors, 224,943 nurses and midwives, and 2,275 pharmacists.[57]

Brain drain is the "academic hemorrhagic syndrome" that has not only left West Africa "immunocompromised" but has contributed greatly to the vulnerability of the sub-region during the Ebola (viral hemorrhagic fever) outbreaks.[60-62] Indeed, brain drain is the "hemorrhagic endemic" before the Ebola hemorrhagic fever epidemic in West Africa.[61,62] There is no way a society can survive with reduced numbers of qualified doctors with such a colossal disease as Ebola. It is no wonder that it did not take an eye's blink before Ebola outran the capacity of the West African medical team.[63] Unfortunately, West Africa witnessed both brain drain and "Ebola drain."

While the former led to the exodus of West African health workers abroad, the latter led some of the remaining West African health workers to their untimely deaths.[53,61-63] Of course, both resulted in dearth of health workers in the West Africa sub-regions.[53,60-63]

Malfunctioning Health facilities: Even before the Ebola outbreaks in West Africa, the health-care delivery system had been neglected because of social conflicts, wars, corruption, bribery, poor governance, and national economic debts.[28] Life expectancy in Liberia, Guinea, Nigeria, and Sierra Leone are respectively 62, 58, 54, and 46 years.[18,57] Most West African public health facilities do not have enough beds, medications, or functioning medical equipment.[64] There are many outdated instruments that have outlived their functions and relevance.[18,57]

Insufficient health centers: In most countries in West Africa, health facilities are concentrated in the cities and urban areas with little or no attention being paid to those in the sub-urban areas or villages.[18,57] It is a major problem for the village-dwellers to bring their sick ones to the nearby health centers.[65] The primary factors responsible for the scanty number of health facilities in the country side, beside the insufficient number of health workers, are the lack of incentive, materials availability, and governmental negligence.[28,66] The hospital bed density in Guinea, Liberia, Nigeria, and Sierra Leone is 0.3 beds/1000 population, 0.8 beds/1000 population, 0.53 beds/1000 population, and 0.4 beds/1000 population respectively.[18]

Lack of health insurance: The concept of health insurance is still very new to many parts of West Africa sub-region, so the majority of patients pay from their pockets.[67] In those situations where patients do not have enough finances or assistance from family members, their health and lives may be compromised.[67] No one can gainsay the importance of health insurance in such a society. Unfortunately health insurance policies are not considered as paramount by most of the West African sub-regional health planners and policymakers.[28]

Low GDP on health: In 2010, Government expenditure on health from the national budget in Guinea, Liberia, Nigeria, and Sierra Leone was 6.8%, 11.1%, 5.7%, and 11.7% respectively [68]. In the same year the per capita expenditure on health in these West African nations was $10, $8, $21, and $10 respectively.[68] This is a far cry from the Abuja commitment that stipulated that 15% of the national budget must be on health.[68]

Traditional medicinal practitioners: From time immemorial, traditional healers have been very active on the African continent.[69] When Africans are sick, most of them first consult the traditional healers before the modern medical providers.[69] African traditional healers consult spirits through incantation, divination, or via mediums.[33] The sick person and the family that attends them almost always have faith in the traditional healers, and believe every word that comes from them.[69] If the traditional healers tell them not to go to the hospital they will not go, If he/she tells them not to tell anyone about the illness, they will not tell.[69] Even after the person dies, the family may still consult the traditional healer to learn what the deceased family member desires, or to know the will or testament of the person.[20,21] So the traditional healer will convey to them the message from the deceased person.[20,21] It is believed that through the traditional medium consultant, the deceased person will inform them how the burial will go, type of color of cloth to be worn during the burial, and what not be done during the burial.[21] If the deceased said the remains should not be cremated the family will comply.[21] According to the International Development Research Centre (IDRC), about 85% of the Sub-Saharan Africa population frequently engage in the services of the traditional medicinal practitioners for primary health care.[70,71]

Nutrition

Unbalanced diet: The staple foods of most West African countries are composed primarily of carbohydrates--a factor that has been implicated in the predisposition to malnutrition.[72,73] Africans believe that you need energy to do most of the manual and unskilled labor in which the majority of them are engaged.[74] It is typical in the West African home to see people eating a whole bowl of carbohydrate such as rice, cassava (cooked), or garri (processed from cassava) with meager amounts of protein in the form of dry meat, fish, or home-grown chicken.[75] Even though most West African people live in an agricultural sector[76] the unfortunate situation is that they would rather sell the best of their farm produce for money than to eat it for their own nutrition. In African culture, the pyramid of food importance is that the head of the family must be given the best part of the food, then follows by the mother, and lastly the children.[77] In certain cases where there are many visitors, if the food being reserved for the guests is not enough, the mother of the home may sacrifice what could have been for her and the children to give to the guests. This type of family food distribution places the women and the children at a very disadvantageous and vulnerable position, hence the prevalence of malnutrition among women, pregnant women, and children.[76, 77]

Bat-eaters: Many families cannot afford to buy meat in most parts of West Africa.[78] Since meat is scarce some people will go for whatever that is animal or animal-like—including chasing after bats.[79] Hence, they scout for bats from caves to coasts and from trees to attics. In the course of hunting for bats some of them may be injured or bitten, and if the bat has a zoonotic disease the human may be infected.[79]

Bush-meat eaters: When you make mention of bush-meat most people will ask you if you are from Africa![79] Of course, there is no doubt that from one part of Africa to another, bush meat is very popular.[79] In major cities or bus-stops, one can easily see the bush-meat sellers promoting it, or see it hanged on the display.[79,80] In most cases, people do not know the conditions of these bush meat, whether they were live animal that were recently killed, or animals that had died many days before someone brought them for sale.[79-81] A lot of diseases such as typhoid fever and zoonotic diseases have been attributed to eating of bush meat in Africa.[81]

Compromised immunity: Even in a pre-disease state some West Africans already have a compromised immunity due to malnutrition.[82] The compromised immune status makes them vulnerable to various kinds of diseases.[83] The prevalence of chronic diseases such as diabetes, AIDS, sickle cell disease and others also affects the immune status of the West Africans--even before the outbreak of Ebola--thus making them more vulnerable.[84-86]

Poor Road infrastructures

The roads in West Africa sub-region are in highly deplorable conditions. There are potholes here and there and many abandoned road projects.[87] This is not only a problem for motorists that must miss gainful employment while fixing broken vehicles, but creating additional havoc for transportation of patients to hospitals or health centers and transferring them from the referring center to specialty centers.[87,88] We were in Africa recently and I and my wife suffered from what we called "road-induced syndrome" which included generalized body ache, neck pain, numbness, nausea, stuffy nose, and vertigo. Because the road was untarred it was dusty and contained bumps and uneven topography. Transportation of sick people, or referring them from one place to another is often a difficult experience—even sometimes complicating the medical problem. In some West African countries where I previously worked the stories of poor roads were similar, I remembered when family members told me how they had to carry sick people on locally made stretchers on their shoulders or backs. They would stop and rest many times before they got to the "bus stop" where vehicle picked them up. It was not an easy thing for both the sick ones and the family members. The poor road infrastructures in West Africa have also been implicated in the majority of the motor vehicle accidents.[89]

Poor Social amenities

Water: Access to potable water is still a nightmare in most parts of West Africa sub-region.[90] In 2012, about 25.2%, 25.4%, 36%, and 36.9% of the populations in Guinea, Liberia, Nigeria, and Sierra Leone respectively had no accessibility to good drinking water.[18] Likewise, the populations in Guinea, Liberia, Nigeria, and Sierra Leone that have no access to proper sanitation facility are 81.1%, 83.2%, 72.2%, and 87% respectively.[18] The water sources in West Africa include tap water or treated water, springs, streams, rain, ponds, dams, and rivers.[91] See Table 4.

Table 4: West Africa and Water and Sanitation

Country	Lack of good water (%)	Lack of good sanitation %
Guinea	25.2	81.1
Liberia	25.4	83.2
Mali	32.8	78.1
Nigeria	36	72.2
Senegal	25.9	48.1
Sierra Leone	36.9	87
Average	30.4	75

Communication: The advent of mobile technology has really revolutionized communication in the West African society in spite of poor coverage by some of the service providers.[88, 92]

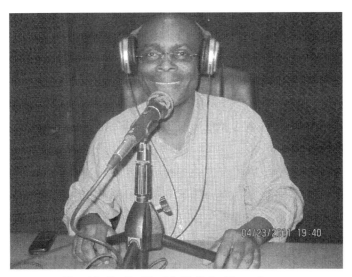

Fig. 12: Radio Health Talk in Sierra Leone

In Guinea, there are 18,000 landline subscribers (0.2% of the population), 4.8 million cellular phone users (41% of the population), 95,000 internet users (0.8% of the population), one government controlled television station with local access, and about 12 radio stations.[18] In Liberia, about 3200 landline subscribers (0.7% of the population) with 2.4 million mobile phone users (56% of the population), 20,000 internet users (0.5% of the population), 4 television stations and 40 radio stations.[18] Nigeria has 418,200 landline phone subscribers (0.2% of the population), 112.8 million mobile phone users (65% of the population), 44 million internet users (25% of the population), about 200 television stations, and over 60 radio stations, while Sierra Leone can only boast of 18,000 landline phone subscribers (0.3% of the population), 2.2 million cellular phone users (36% of the population), 14,900 internet users (0.2% of the population), 3 television stations, and 25 radio stations.[18] The higher the number of functional broadcasting media, the faster the information dissemination and the more populations that will be reached.[18,88,92] Communication is very vital to dissemination of news about any communicable diseases or outbreaks.[92] See table 5.

Table 5: West African Countries and Communications

Country	Landline (%)	Cell Phone (%)	Internet (%)
Guinea	0.2	41	0.8
Liberia	0.7	56	0.5
Mali	0.7	88.8	2
Nigeria	0.2	65	25
Senegal	2.5	84.1	13.3
Sierra Leone	0.3	36	2
Average	0.8	61.8	7.3

Lack of social security system: When the bread winners in Africa are quarantined or isolated because of Ebola, his or her major worries are not about the disease but about those he or she is providing food for. There is no social security system in most countries in West Africa sub-region, resulting in the majority of the population economically vulnerable. According to the International Labor Organization (ILO), only about 10% of the working population has some form of social security coverage in the sub-Saharan Africa.[93] Since there is no financial security for most people, they live from hands to mouth on a meager income. Without this social security system in West Africa, the socio-economic future of large number of the population is bleak.[94]

Chapter Five
West African Intra-Ebola Situation

Poor preparation

Lack of promptly designated isolation centers: It took a while before it finally dawned on the people of West Africa sub-region that Ebola had entered our sub-region uninvited and that we must wage a relentless war against it.[95] There was no preparation against the possible arrival of some catastrophic communicable disease such as Ebola in spite of the fact that Ebola has been around in East Africa since 1976.[96,97] It is sad to say that most countries in the sub-region major in "fire brigade approach" to castrophies, but minor in anticipated preparation.[97] The saddest of it all is that these countries in the West Africa sub-region depend more on outside powers to solve their problems[98,99] but do not like to listen and follow the advice of these same powers for ensuring transparency, accountability, and "follow-through-economic" plans.[100] Prior to the outbreaks, most hospitals in the sub-region had no isolation wards or quarantine rooms which are very germane to curbing Ebola spread.[101]

Deficient infectious disease training: The Ebola outbreaks in West Africa did not only over-power the region from the outset, but also revealed how deficient and superficial the training on infectious diseases was.[96] The limited extent of medical training necessary to recognize and manage disease through treatment or referral is not only applicable to common diseases, but to rare ones as well.[102] There is no iota of doubt that if there had been adequate training and sufficient preparation regarding tropical infectious diseases, especially those that are life-threatening, the morbidity, mortality and fatality rates could have been different.[103-105]

Lack of resources

Lack of personal protective equipment (PPE): The PPE needed for health workers against Ebola includes long gloves, a face mask, fluid-resistant, full body covering gowns, goggles (or face shield), booties, and hoods.[1, 2, 6] These are special kinds of PPE that do not allow skin exposure.[6, 106,107] It is often advised to use double gloves when necessary to ensure that there is no accidental glove break or glove-factory failure. Those that are involved in burying Ebola victims must also wear long, fluid-resistant "Ebola" boots as well.[106] The correct donning (putting on) and doffing (putting off) of PPE is as importance as having the correct fluid-impermeable full-body covering gowns.[1,6,107]

Insufficient fund: Due to lack of adequate preparation and the small allocation from the national GDP on health, there were no enough funds to fight Ebola outbreaks in West Africa.[108] The most appalling thing is that the largest portion of the money allocated to procure the required PPE for the health workers and blood-borne pathogen kits for hospitals did not reach the place where it was needed.[109] The majority of the countries in West Africa rely solely on foreign aid for almost all aspects of the national budgets.[28] According to Dr. Peter Piot (who discovered Ebola in 1976) in his interview with the BBC World Service in 2014, "We shouldn't forget that this is a disease of poverty, of dysfunctional health systems - and of distrust."[4]

Politico-security instability

West Africa countries are plagued by unstable governments and security concerns, either from within the country itself, or from neighboring countries.[110,111] In recent times, the menace of terrorist groups is growing in the sub-region and increasingly becoming a source of worries to everyone.[112,113] The terrorist groups in Mali and northern Nigeria, (just to mention but few) are not only murdering, maiming, kidnapping, and looting, but constitute as well, national economic woes, fears, and regional entropy.[114,115] There are both internal and external displacements of civilians, most of whom are women, children, elderly, and other vulnerable people in the society.[116,117] With political instability and uncertainty come the loss of personal freedom, economic means and properties, and the escalation of civil and social conflicts that also compromise health and immunity.[118]

Conflicting Ebola message

At the outset there was no clear message on how to diagnose, treat, and prevent Ebola.[109] It really caught the West Africa sub-region off its guard (if at all there was any guard in place before) for there were very few standard laboratories for confirmatory diagnosis.[119] As pointed out by Dr. Peter Piot, the same posters containing Ebola health education messages indicating that there was no cure for Ebola instructed infected people to go to Ebola treatment centers. This was very confusing to the general public.[120] Since Ebola in the early stages of the disease can present as malaria or typhoid fever, which are very common in the sub-region, it led to a time lag before it was finally recognized that it was not just a surge in malaria and typhoid fever cases but an entirely new disease outbreak – Ebola.[2]

Ebola outbreak was very new to the sub-region and most health practitioners had only scantily read about it in textbooks--believing that it was confined to East Africa, and assuming that they would never come across an Ebola case during their lifetime practice. Therefore, refreshing courses were needed to readily combat the disease.[121] Unfortunately, Ebola, for the first time, left the borders of the East Africa and came to the West Africa sub-region uninvited. There it created in a short time greater havoc than it had in all the years combined in the Eastern part of Africa. In truth, this is Ebola without respect for borders! The big lesson is this, what affects anywhere can affect everywhere!

False traditional health attendant claims

In most parts of West Africa traditional healers fill in the gap resulting from insufficient numbers of qualified medical personnel. This is especially true in the remote villages where qualified health workers are very reluctant to go.[122] Most of these remote villages share borders with other neighboring countries, making them more vulnerable to inter-border communicable diseases.[123,124] Most of the border villages are neglected by the central governments, either due to border disputes or lack of funds.[28] There are some village dwellers that have no access at all to the modern health-care delivery system--due to poverty, or to dependence upon traditional healers.[122,125] There is no doubt that it takes many more years to formally train a doctor than to train a traditional healer who inherits his practice from the family--and receiving only informal training. To the average traditional healer the presentation and treatment of Ebola is no different than other febrile illnesses. Some traditional healers also believe that the source of disease is the result of someone in the family or neighborhood bewitching the sick person.[122] This then may lead to name-calling--thus creating or furthering a rift, conflict, and mistrust in the family.[126] Because of issues of bewitching or spell-casting, traditional healers often hide patients in their homes, even advising the patients and families that this kind of sickness is not good for hospitals.[126,127] The traditional healers do not use the barrier methods or wash their hands after coming in contact with patients, thus enhancing the spread of communicable diseases like Ebola.[126,128] Because traditional healers do not use laboratory tools to diagnose Ebola they do not know what Ebola really is and thus end up in denying the existence of it.[126,128] Most traditional healers depend on traditional African healing practice for their livelihoods, so they do not always admit that there are diseases they do not know of or cannot cure.[129] Many traditional healers that have large families so they are compelled to lay claim to knowing almost everything in order to provide for their families. Many people thought that the Liberian that brought EVD to Nigeria actually traveled to Nigeria with the hope of seeking help from the miracle-healer or faith-healer.[130, 131] Unfortunately, he collapsed at the Murtala Mohammed Airport, Lagos, Nigeria, and was taken to the First Consultant Hospital, Lagos. He was resuscitated and was asked to wait for his laboratory results which also included Ebola test.[131] According to the BBC news, Dr. Benjamin Ohiaeri, the medical director of First Consultant Hospital, said, "Immediately, he was very aggressive. He was more intent on leaving the hospital than anything else." The index patient called his Liberian Embassy in Nigeria and someone from the Liberian Embassy then called and threatened the hospital staff that they would be blacklisted as kidnappers if they did not release the index patient from their hospital; all in an attempt to get him to the miracle-healer before he would attend the ECOWAS conference he came for.[130-132] His blood test proved that he had EVD and was not released but eventually died in the hospital.[131] Culture plays major role in how people often seek for health-care, compliance, and the outcome of health-care management they seek for.[133,134] It is the common saying in Africa that you might succeed in taking Africans out of Africa Continent but you cannot succeed enough to take African tradition (Africa culture, African medicinal belief, voodoo practice, faith-healing, spiritualism, entertainment, resilience, and Africanism) out of their bloodstream.

Lack of faith in Government health message

Because of years of neglect, bribery, corruption, and lack of transparency and accountability there is a lack of trust between the government and the people. This has resulted in anger against the government and its message.[28] Hence the majority of the populace did not believe what the government was talking about concerning Ebola. They believed that it was just another governmental design to get money from the international community.[135,136] Accordingly, people tended to believe that they had become pawns in the hands of the government to attract foreign donations and assistance.[135-137] At first the people did not pay heed to the community preventative health message warning them to avoid such things as eating bats and bush meat, playing with monkeys, overcrowding, touching the dead--and even the reality of Ebola epidemic.[138,139] In addition, families would often hide sick members that had likely been infected with Ebola from health workers, or from going to the Ebola designated centers. Even infected pregnant women with bleeding would claim that they had an abortion instead and giving the true picture of the situation.[135]

Ebola-spread-enhancing cultural practices

Burial ritual

Corpse-washing: Africans are very caring for the dead, and in order to show affection and to prove that the love they have for the person is not diminished even though dead, they continue to give special attention to his/her body.[20,21] They will do a thorough wash and apply perfume and an oily cream to the body of the dead.[20,21] The practice washing the body- and applying the oily cream is not only to demonstrate love, but also because of a deep believe in life after death and the need to preserve the body against early decomposition.[21] It is a common belief in Africa that only those that have committed evil deeds do not deserve corpse-washing, irrespective of the types of death.[21] They do not wear gloves when they are doing body washing and anointing the body of the dead one with oil and perfume.[126] The practice of body washing brings the people into direct contact with body fluids of the dead person, especially when a cut or injury is present, and in case of Ebola, enhances transmission of the deadly disease.[126,140]

Preservation of certain parts: African culture promotes a spiritual link with the ancestors,[141] and one of the ways they ensure that the link is not broken is by preserving certain parts of the body of the dead ones.[21,] This practice may be fading away now but it is still being practiced in some quarters--especially when a powerful individual, chief, or king dies.[21] The survivors may cut the nails, hair, or any other parts of the deceased (corpse) in accordance with the tradition![21] At the coronation of the successor to the vacant stool (throne) these parts will be handed over to him or her.[21] It is a customary belief that by having these parts of the powerful person with them, the spirit of the deceased remains nearby, and when consulted, will answer, since he (she) did not go beyond with all of his (her) parts.[21] If peradventure the dead one contracted Ebola before death, this practice may act as a channel of Ebola spread.

Holding and wailing on the corpse

Naturally, Africans are people of communal culture.[142] They believe in identifying with people whether in time of joy or sorrow, whether in success or suffering.[143] This belief also includes mourning for deceased relatives. If one does not cry or mourn, the society may infer that you somehow contribute to the dead of that person. Typically, African society does not only mourn the dead but also observes the reaction of the relatives or the friends of the dead.[144] The measure of how much you love the dead one is determined by the degree of your wailing, crying, or mourning, and whether or not you were touching the corpse while crying.[21,126] If you cried and did not touch the corpse or hold on to the corpse dearly[145] until the time it was taken away from you, those that came to sympathize with you may, in the future, refer to your indifferent behavior towards the dead as an act of wickedness. No one wants to be labeled as a wicked person in the society so the practice of holding dearly to the corpse while mourning[145] has become entrenched in the African society. Because mourners eventually come in contact with someone that died of Ebola, this practice undoubtedly serves as an avenue for Ebola transmission.[2, 21]

Lack of hygiene

Hygienic practice is poor even after the individual has been in contact with the body fluids of someone with Ebola.[2, 21,146] Hand washing and the use of disinfectants are seldom employed.[126] There is no doubt that Africans want to show how much they love their sick ones by being around them and communicating their love non-verbally by touching the sick. They also consider it as a form of apathy to wash hands after touching their sick loved ones.[126] By washing hands after touching a sick person who has been very close to you, it may be thought that you love the person less because of the sickness. This is unfortunate since one of the most important ways to halt the spread of Ebola is to do hand washing or to use disinfectant lotion.[6]

Eating customs

Because of the ardent African belief and practice of a culture of communion, eating together from the same plate is viewed as a demonstration of togetherness, oneness, and love.[147] Even when the person is sick, Africans still want to eat together with the sick individual in order to convey the idea that sickness does not diminish or limit their love for their sick one.[130] Accordingly, anyone who avoids eating together with the rest of family is viewed as one who is uninterested in, or opposed to maintaining the bond of family unity.[21,126] There is a saying in Africa, "If you eat alone you die alone," so African culture promotes eating together as a family.

Sharing sleeping bed with the sick

The majority of Africans usually sleep together, babies and siblings all sharing the same bed and sleeping with the mother.[149,150] Africans also sleep in the same bed with the sick person in order to care for his/her needs better. They believe that the healthy members of the family are better able to care for the more vulnerable ones that are sick..[21, 126,130] I remembered when I was young and was sick with malaria, my parents used to be on the same bed with me. Africans believe that sleeping with sick one also allows them to monitor the progress of the disease, and in case of complications or worsening of the condition, the healthy family member will be able to alert others to get help more rapidly. However, this practice does involve body contact with the sick and if the person is infected with EVD, this may facilitate Ebola transmission.

Greeting norms

Hugging: Africans have a long tradition of taking long time to greet others.[151] It is believed that the more time you spend in greeting someone the more you show that you love and respect the person.[21,152] This act of greeting also involves hugging each other dearly and closely.[126,152] The general belief is that love is centered in the heart and when one hugs the chest where heart is situated, one is thereby touching the heart of the other--thus signifying the communication of love, compassion, and trust to the other.[153] The greeting will also entail questions regarding the wellbeing of the other, and of the other members of the family.[154] Africans really cherish greetings. Accordingly, they may be exchanged anywhere, everywhere, every time, and anytime.[154] They greet each other in the market places, at the stream while fetching water, on the road when meeting each other, at the farm while working, at religious centers, and in offices.[21,154]

Kissing: In some parts of West Africa sub-region, a greeting is followed by a sign of love by either giving a light lip-kiss or cheek-kiss.[155] In some African cultures, people kiss corpses in a show of respect and reverence for the dead.[140] Though in times past, a handshake was not a usual practice in Africa, but it is very common now.

Living Conditions

Family living together: In the African culture of inclusion and togetherness, there are no cousins, nephews, uncles, or aunts. We only have brothers, sisters, mothers, and fathers.[141] This, we do in order to convey a sense of belonging, oneness, love, and the spirit of "brotherhood, sisterhood, motherhood, or fatherhood."[156] It is not unusual to see in one house or compound great grandparents living in the same place with the grandparents, parents, and young ones.[156] Living together is considered as a clear sign that the family is truly united, assuring that the older generations can easily pass down family values and virtues to the younger generations.[157] The family name and dignity are seen as a big deal in the African society. Africans believe that the "Traditional man is not surrounded by things but by beings."[158] Truly, they may not have money, but they are happy and feel so proud because the family is viewed as the most priceless asset any one can ever have.[159] The younger generations are able to take care of their older generations as aging set in.[160] Most African society does not have special homes for the elderly. Rather, the homes that the older generations have been accustomed to, continue to be their home until they die.[160] However, this practice can easily promote the spread of disease among the family--especially when the disease is infectious such as Ebola or cholera.

Overcrowding

Due to social conflicts, poverty, displacements, unemployment, and family togetherness, overcrowding is a common problem in most parts of the West African sub-region. In fact, it is possible to see an entire household; father, mother, and 2 or 3 children living together in one small room.[161] And whenever someone comes to visit, the same small room will be shared by them all. Overcrowding enhances the spread of communicable diseases such as tuberculosis, Ebola, measles, and others.[162]

Magnanimous norms

Bush meat sharing: Africans by nature are very magnanimous, whatever one has is considered to be for all of us.[163] When a hunter kills an animal (bush meat) it will be shared with his family, friends, and neighbors.[164] Unfortunately, if the animal is infected with disease, it will also endanger all those that partake of it. Infected bush meat has been implicated in the spread of Ebola.[165]

Other food stuff sharing: Africans do not only share bush meat, but also share other food stuff, both plant-based and animal based.[164] During festivals (traditional, religious, or national), Africans will cook food and share with others, and others will also share with you.[166] When someone dies, Africans will celebrate the life of that person, especially if the person was old or held an important position in life, by merry making (eating, drinking, and partying).[167,168] As a matter of fact, no one goes hungry during time of festivities. Unfortunately, food-borne diseases can easily be transmitted by this practice.

Anti-sociocultural consideration of Ebola isolation: Because of the communal cultural practice of the African society, [156] isolating a sick person because of Ebola is viewed as anti-social and lacking empathy. They love to care for the sick and when someone is isolated, their access to the sick one is restricted. Traditionally, Africans feel that everyone except those that have done evil deserve care when they are sick.[21] Isolation is considered culturally as depriving, and denying the sick person of the human care and love they need.[126] When someone is sick in Africa and admitted in the hospital, almost everyone, from the young to the old, friends and foes, male and female, will come to visit during the visiting hours. They believe that when the sick person sees how many come to visit them, they will realize how much they are loved and valued and will be encouraged to fight for life, and return back from illness.[130] Likewise, when an ill person does not see anyone visiting them, it may appear to them that they are not wanted around any longer, leading them to conclude that dying is probably better than living.[21] One of the major challenges I faced during the years I worked in Nigeria, Liberia, The Gambia, and Sierra Leone was the ability to covey the importance of isolation to patient relatives. Even after performing operations on patients, families and relatives wanted to see and be around the person immediately. This posed serious challenges for conveying the message that I knew how much they loved the person and how great the desire to be around them, but at this point in time the patient needed time to recover from the anesthetic effects. Some people liked the explanation while to others my explanation did not go so well. Of course, in case of communicable diseases, isolation is not an option but one of the cardinal standards of management.[1,2] Many families resisted isolation, or even hid their infected ones from the health workers out of fear of being isolated. There were instances where relatives broke into the isolation unit in Liberia, forcefully taking their isolated, infected, family members away.[169] This problem added to the uncontrollable spread of Ebola in these West African countries.[170]

Cultural importance of burial ground or cemetery

Social unacceptability of cremation: In African culture, cremation is not socially acceptable for anyone (except those that have committed a heinous or nefarious activity).[171] Yet, in order to prevent the spread of the Ebola virus via the transmission of body fluids, and to eradicate the Ebola virus, cremation has become the gold standard of practice for the disposal of the infected corpse.[1,2] Unfortunately, this standard practice is causing an "Ebola-eradication cultural shock" to the West African society.[172] Surviving family members are faced with the difficult decision of whether to cooperate with the authorities and give their loved one(s) over for cremation, or of resisting those authorities and burying the loved one(s) with all the traditional rites and rituals, and thereby continue to spread Ebola in the community. It is a real cultural conflict and cultural dilemma that the people face.

Social discrimination if family burial site is unknown or if the burial rite is undone: A great deal of emphasis is placed on knowing where the family member is buried so as to be able to perform the traditional burial rites at the burial site.[177] Major cultural confusion arises when African families do not know the location or have access to the burial sites of their deceased family or loved ones.[21] Often, if there is conflict or misunderstanding between one family and another, one ridicules the other if the accused family does not know where the deceased family member is buried--or if a traditional burial has not been performed.[21,178] This kind of social discrimination[179] is common in the closed African society. Surely word goes around and the individual or the family may become objects of ridicule. Even the Ebola burial teams are being stigmatized.[178]

Bat

Food: In some parts of West Africa, bats are considered to be delicious bush meat.[180] Most food and eating practices in West Africa are generational. Therefore, telling someone to desist from eating bats or certain other foods will be met with resistance.[21] In fact they may tell you that their grandfather ate it and lived to become a very old man. Since the practice of eating bats is often considered as having a traditional connotation it may be very difficult to wean the people from it.

Another factor driving people to eat bats is the problem of poverty. Bat meat may be available as a substitute when people cannot afford other types of meat. According to the World Bank 2011 economic report, the poverty headcount ratio at $1.25 a day of Sub-Saharan Africa was 46.8%.[183] (See figure 13).

Bats are also known to be a reservoir for other zoonotic diseases apart from Ebola.[181, 182] An infected bat bite can result in Ebola, rabies or one of a number of other life-threatening diseases [181]

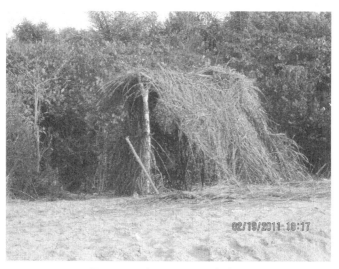

Fig. 13: A Temporary Shelter

Traditional medicinal importance: Since it is a general belief in Africa that bats sleep during the day time and do not sleep at night, they are sometimes used medicinally to help keep people awake when hunting during the night, serving as a night-watch or neighborhood night guide, or some other such activity. Apart from being used as an antidote to sleepiness, bats may be used to induce love, or as charms for bringing good luck.[184] "Bat magic" (folk medicine) may be prescribed to give good vision to hunters so that they will always hit the target without missing it.[184] The traditional African healers also use bats for those with paralysis or nerve problems.[21] Scientifically, it had been demonstrated that the vampire bat has plasminogen activator DSPA-alpha-1 (desmoteplase) that functions as a thrombolytic drug for individual with ischemic stroke.[185,186] Bats are also used to restore hair in male baldness.[180,186]

Traditional religion: In traditional African religion, since bats are different from other animals or birds, they are considered as special creatures.[184] The adoration giving to bats by the traditional African religionists is borne out of the fact that other creatures sleep with their heads up but that bats sleep with the heads down, suggesting that they may possess qualities that other creatures do not have.[187] The traditional African religionists also saw another distinguishing feature in bats that are not shared by other creatures. Bats possess both animal and bird characteristics.[187] Out of fear for the god or goddess that made bats, African traditionalists revere that deity so that he/she will not at any point in time turn their lives into that of a bat, which is characterized by ambiguity.[187] Accordingly, in Nigerian Yoruba traditional life, when someone has a dubious character, the saying goes, "He/she is neither animal nor bird, just like a bat." It means no one can really define or know his/her true character or identity.

Sharing of deceased personal belongings: Africans believe that when a family member dies and has not committed any heinous activity, the belongings must be shared.[21,33,34,188] But in case of a family with nefarious activity that dies, his or her belongings will be burned and not be used.[21] The unfortunate thing about this practice of sharing the deceased belongings is that it may aid the transmission of contagious disease, including the Ebola virus.

Stealing of Ebola isolation materials: The high level of unemployment and poverty in the West Africa sub-region tempted the youth to view Ebola isolation wards as a sign of luxury. Since most of them slept without beds and mattresses, a group of them decided to break in and steal the materials from the isolation wards in Liberia.[189] Of course, these were materials that had been contaminated with Ebola virus--all of which aided the spread of Ebola.[190]

Power of money and Position

The sick Liberian man that brought Ebola to Nigeria was aware that he could not travel to another country because of restrictions on any sick person from traveling outside of Liberia[130,131] He also knew that as long as he could get to the airport he could bribe his way out,[130] because he knew bribery and corruption is endemic at the sea and air ports.[191] The man was highly placed in the government so he was able to use his position to work his way out.[130]

Even the Ebola burial teams were bribed by the Ebola corpse families in order for these families to perform traditional burial rites on those Ebola-infected corpses.[192]

Ebola fraud

Because of poverty and lack of transparency, and since ample financial assistance was coming to Africa from the international community, some people used the Ebola crisis to enrich themselves by engaging in fraudulent activities.[193] So, there were ghost workers and fake projects in order to divert the money meant for Ebola crisis to the private purse, thereby increasing the difficulty of controlling the disease in the sub-region.[193]

Ebola Diagnostic Difficulty

Mimic other diseases: Ebola cannot be accurately diagnosed clinically without proper laboratory investigations.[1,2] It is very easy to mistake Ebola for malaria fever and/or typhoid fever, and these two diseases are very common in the West Africa sub-region.[194]

Wrong diagnosis: Because the list of differential diagnosis for Ebola is very long, the probability of incorrectly diagnosing Ebola is high.[195] This was especially true at the beginning of the outbreaks when the index of suspicion of Ebola was very low. [196]

Lack of well-equipped laboratory: The problem was not only the lack of well-equipped laboratories in the sub-region, but the number of qualified laboratory scientists that specialize in Ebola laboratory investigations was also very limited.[197] Most laboratory science training in West Africa does not include Ebola. The curriculum and training are centered on "common things that occur commonly" such as malaria parasites, helminthes, protozoa, sickle cell prep, and widal test.[198,199]

Lengthy days before diagnostic results: It takes a minimum of about 3 days after exposure to Ebola before the virus in the blood can reach a detectable level.[1,2] Most health centers in the sub-region depend on the central laboratory for their diagnostic results which are at times are very far from the health centers. This fact creates a significant time lag in obtaining the laboratory results.[199]

Other diseases' negligence

The attention given to the Ebola outbreak has had a major negative impact upon other prevailing health care needs in West Africa. For example, under-5 malnutrition, diarrhea, malaria, and obstetrical complications in the sub-region have suffered greatly by the diversion of financial resources to fund the Ebola fight.[200] UNFPA estimated that 800,000 women will give birth in 2015 in Guinea, Liberia, and Sierra Leone, but about 120,000 of them would die from lack of emergency obstetrical care because most of these countries' health services have been diverted toward the Ebola response.[201] Other non-Ebola care services are also lagging behind, especially in Sierra Leone where only 20% of the 10,000 HIV patients on anti-retroviral treatments are currently receiving the medication for lack of health personnel that have been called upon to fight the Ebola war.[201]

Travel restrictions, quarantine

In order to contain the spread of Ebola from the West African hotspots, travel restrictions and quarantine were employed to contain the outbreaks.[11] Since Ebola has an incubation period of about 21 days, the duration of quarantine for Ebola is set at 21 days.[1, 2] This measure is used, not only to determine if the person has contracted the disease but, also to prevent spreading it to others.[1,2]

School closure

In order to prevent the spread of Ebola in schools, the various governments in the Ebola affected countries in West Africa mandated school closures[202]. It was a just cause in the Ebola war since the lives of the future generations could be affected by this outbreak. Pupils and students could easily transmit it among themselves, to teachers, and other members of their households.[202]

Ebola screening

Port of entry and exit: Neighboring countries to the Ebola-stricken West Africa sub-region not only imposed travel bans, but also screened those that were coming or traveling out of their nations--an effort to enhance early detection.[203, 204] Health workers at the port of entry and exit, in addition to filling out the Ebola screening forms, used screening thermometers to record the temperature of.[11, 203]

Other screening measures put were in place to promote early detection on Ebola in the countryside.[205] Those schools for which the government did not mandate closure utilized screening of their students in the morning when students came from homes and in the afternoon before the schools were closed for that day.[206]

Local unscientific preventive measures

High salt solution ingestion: Ebola fear gripped most people in the West Africa sub-region, especially when the health message also included the understanding that "Ebola has no cure." In response, various practices arose in an attempt to avoid contracting Ebola. One of these employed the drinking of high-salt solutions.[207,208] The question on every lip was, why are people using high salt solution to prevent Ebola? Where did they get the idea of using high salt solution to prevent Ebola? Why did they decide to use high salt solution and not low salt solution? I was as curious as others to know the rationale for the practice. One of the salient properties and uses of salt is as a preservative. Those that were using high salt solutions in the attempt to prevent Ebola had in mind that the preservative property of salt would preserve their blood system and body from attack by Ebola. They also believed that the higher the salt concentration of the solution, the greater the power of preservation. That was the reason why they did not use low salt solution, thinking that it would be too weak to fight a strong disease like Ebola that had been killing without discrimination. Unfortunately, the high salt (hypertonic) solution can also result in fever, hypervolemia, and depletion of intracellular fluid.[209] (See figure 14). In case of those with high blood pressure (hypertension), a condition that is very common among the black African populations, it would tend to exacerbate the medical condition.[210] One of my cousins in Nigeria told me how she almost died as a result of following the example of others in drinking the high salt solution. There is no clinical evidence supporting the claim that high salt solution could prevent anyone from contracting Ebola.[211, 212]

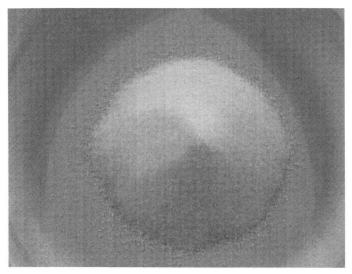

Fig. 14: Table Salt

High Bitter kola nut consumption: Since there is no definitive or specific care for Ebola except for palliative and symptomatic treatment, the people were constantly seeking for alternative remedies to prevent contracting the disease.[215] One of these was the kola nut. Garcinia kola is one of the folk medicines used for fever, cold, and possibly boosting one's immunity.[215,216] Since people believed that bitter kola nut had preventive properties against Ebola, there was a sudden surge in the local sale of bitter kola nut (Garcinia kola) (see figure 15). As a result, as demand exceeded supply, the sellers of the bitter kola nut quickly ran out of stocks—and the corresponding high profits.[216] One will not hesitate to ask, why people would think that bitter kola nut has preventive functions against Ebola? Why not other kola nuts that are not bitter? The answer I got from some friends in Nigeria that ate the bitter kola nut was, "Bitter kola nut is bitter as the name suggests. Eating it will make our blood to be too bitter for Ebola to feed on." There is a statement in Africa one may make to someone one thinks might harm them, "My blood is bitter," meaning you cannot harm me as long as my blood is bitter. They also believe that sweet things encourage microbes to grow. Therefore, if they continue to eat a lot of bitter kola nuts, they think their blood would be bitter and thus would not serve as a culture media for Ebola to grow or thrive in. Of course there is no scientific evidence or support for this.[215]

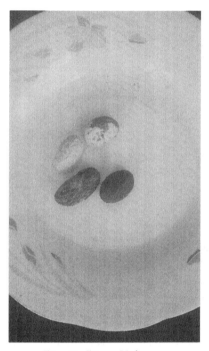

Fig. 15: Bitter Kola nut

Media role

The media played a very significant role in not only creating sensational news about Ebola in the West Africa sub-region, but in drawing the attention of the world to what was happening in a previously non-Ebola designated zone.[217,218] Prior to the 2014 Ebola outbreaks, Ebola had been geographically restricted to East Africa, but for the first time it left its usual domain and gained entrance into the newfound West Africa sub-region.[219,220] The media also mobilized the world to donate, send medical teams, PPE, and other necessary logistics to fight the outbreaks.[221] Some might argue that the media over-emphasized the negative side of the news regarding the lack of effective Ebola treatment, lack of vaccines, and hope of cure, and thereby contributed to the fear and panic that resulted.[217,218] The bottom line is that the media also promoted the preventive aspects and gave the "current situation and dire need" of the Ebola war in the West Africa[222] that was regularly plighted by social conflicts and wars.[28]

Assistance

United Nations (UN): The UN initiated a global Ebola response that put countries together to donate and send humanitarian aid, and medical teams to the mostly affected West African states.[223] Other UN organizations such as UNDP, UNFPA, and Food and Agriculture Organization (FAO) also galvanized necessary resources to help the affected West African countries.[224,225] FAO announced at the beginning of this year (2015) that Guinea, Liberia, and Sierra Leone will each receive $500,000 assistance to ameliorate Ebola-induced food insecurity that affects households and livelihoods of farmers and others in rural settlements. The funds, to be distributed over a 12-month period, would cover about 7,500 households or 45,000 people in the badly affected countries.[223]

Ebola virus might be used in bioterrorism, a situation that could be very devastating. Certainly, a global effort should be coordinated to prevent the virus from falling into the hands of terrorists.[59]

United States of America (USA): Even though the President of the United States, Barack Obama, in a speech delivered on February 11, 2015, did not specifically state "mission accomplished," did indicate that he believed that since the Ebola was being observed as scaling down, by the end of April, 2015, most of the 1,300 US troops that had been working in Liberia for the past 5 months could return to their home bases.[226] According to US defense officials, The Pentagon would still like to keep about 100 service members in Liberia to strengthen "disease preparedness and surveillance capacity."[226] The returnees would still undergo the 21-day quarantine procedures with a self-controlled monitoring process, looking especially for fever and any other tale-telling symptoms that might suggest infectious disease.[226-228] Whenever any of these symptoms might appear, the individual is to report immediately for admission and isolation, and the beginning of supportive treatment--acknowledging the fact that early detection and prompt treatment are very germane to high chances of survival of Ebola disease.[226-228] Liberia and the US have a long history of interaction since Liberia was founded by the freed slaves that were brought from the US in 1820 and declared independence in 1847.[229]

United Kingdom (UK): The United Kingdom action plan to defeat Ebola in Sierra Leone included providing 100 million Great Britain Pound Sterling that would provide for 700 Ebola treatment beds and Ebola treatment facilities and support for social mobilization. This included contact tracing, burial services, commodity and community level care, and to pay national and international Ebola-related staff.[230]

Archeologically, Sierra Leone has been inhabited for at least 2,500 years. It had its first contact with the European Portuguese in 1462.[231] Freed slaves were brought in by the UK in the years of 1787 and 1792. From the year 1800 until 1960 Sierra Leone was colonized by the UK, and in 1961 she was granted independence.[231]

France: France not only built Ebola treatment centers in Guinea, but French President, Francois Hollande, visited in November 2014. While there he announced that France would be committing 100 million euros to Guinea with which to establish treatment and preventive measures to fight Ebola outbreaks.[232] In 1891, France declared Guinea to be her colony. She regained her independence in 1958.[233]

Economic Community of West Africa States (ECOWAS): The West African Health Organization (WAHO) is saddled with the responsibility by the ECOWAS to synchronize and coordinate cross-border activities that included, "surveillance, case management and contact tracing, harmonization of communication strategies, sharing of logistic information and resources, and supervision and evaluation of interventions."[234] Other deliberated actions included "developing and implementing control plans for preparedness and response, increased awareness on individual and collective protection measures, social mobilization, personnel training, strengthening Ebola virus disease surveillance and early warning in airports, ports, gathering places at border posts and at all health care units."[19,234] ECOWAS efforts also involved in the provision of PPE, medicines, health personnel manpower, non-health personnel staff, implementation of synchronized cross-border interventions, and strengthening of laboratory services.[19,234]

African Union (AU): The African Union responded to the Ebola outbreaks in West Africa by forming African Union Support to Ebola Outbreak in West Africa (ASEOWA) to manage 100 beds in Liberia, 100 beds in Sierra Leone, two Ebola treatment units (ETU) in Guinea, and to provide epidemiological support and medical training to medical staff in the affected countries.[235] AU donated about 1.1 million dollars to fighting Ebola outbreak in West Africa.[235]

World Bank: The World Bank Group mobilized nearly $1 billion in financing for the countries hardest hit by the Ebola crisis.[13] This included $518 million from IDA, the World Bank Group's fund for the poorest countries for the emergency response, and at least $450 million from IFC, a member of the World Bank Group, to enable trade, investment, and employment in Guinea, Liberia, and Sierra Leone.[13]

Non-Governmental Organization (NGO): Both local and international non-governmental not-for-profit, or charity organizations, were involved in the fight against Ebola outbreaks in West Africa.[236] They provided medical personnel, humanitarian aids, logistics, funds, medicine, and non-medical personnel. The prominent international NGOs included, but were not limit to, Medecins Sans Frontieres (MSF) (doctors without borders), Adventist Development and Relief Agency (ADRA), Bill and Melinda Gates Foundation, and the Catholic Relief Services. Together, these organizations have provided a major contribution toward the control of the Ebola epidemic.[237]

MSF has been involved in managing Ebola outbreaks in East Africa and thus has an age-long experience and protocols in managing Ebola disease and outbreaks.[238] Since March of 2014 when it was first announced that Ebola broke out in Guinea, MSF's has been in the forefront.[16] In addition to Guinea, MSF is also actively involved in the Ebola management in Liberia, Mali, and Sierra Leone.[239] The capacity of MSF in the West Africa sub-region includes 325 international, and about 4150 national locally hired staff, 8 Ebola case management centers (CMCs), 650 beds in isolation, and 1 transit center.[16] As of the time of this writing, MSF had admitted more than 8,100 patients. Of these, about 4,960 were confirmed Ebola cases, of which more than 2,300 survived.[16] MSF has shipped over 1,400 tons of supplies to the affected West African countries.[16] Dr. Armand Sprecher,

Public Health Specialist at MSF, spoke about MSF approaches to managing Ebola. These include symptomatic care, supportive care, presumptive care, nutritional support, and psychosocial counseling.[16] Symptomatic care consists of providing medication to bring the fever down, relieve pain, and to stop vomiting and diarrhea.[16,240] In MSF supportive care, fluid loss is replaced, either through oral rehydration if patient is stable and can tolerate, or with intravenous fluid if patient is in an unstable condition or vomiting.[16,240] Presumptive care involves treating any co-morbid diseases such as malaria, typhoid, shigellosis, and others, since these diseases if untreated can further compromise a patient's immune status and worsen the Ebola condition.[1,2,16] Nutritional support includes the provision of vitamins and therapeutic foods to ensure that patients have balanced diets to help build up the body immunity.[16] Most of them might have had a compromised nutritional status even before the Ebola attack.[16] In helping the patients and families to deal with the Ebola-induced psychological trauma, MSF also provides psychosocial counseling.[16]

Table 6: March 25, 2014-March 29, 2015 Ebola Distribution

Country	Region	Types	Cases	Deaths	Fatality
Guinea	W. Africa	Zaire virus	3492	2314	66.3%
Liberia	W. Africa	Zaire virus	9712	4432	45.6%
Mali	W. Africa	Zaire virus	8	6	75%
Nigeria	W. Africa	Zaire virus	20	8	40%
Senegal	W. Africa	Zaire virus	1	0	0%
Sierra Leone	W. Africa	Zaire virus	11974	3799	31.7%
Spain	EU	Zaire virus	1	0	0%
UK	EU	Zaire virus	1	0	0%
USA	N. America	Zaire virus	4	1	25%

Ebola distribution[15]

Chapter Six
West African Post-Ebola State

Depletion of the meagre health resources

It did not take long after Ebola was discovered in West Africa before it became clear to the whole world that not only was the West Africa sub-region un-prepared for any eventuality, but that it did not even have enough resources to see them through the immediate problem.[241] The naked truth is that whatever health infrastructures and resources the West Africa sub-region had prior to Ebola, the most seriously affected countries have nothing left anymore.[242] The unfortunate situation is that since their available meagre resources were expended in fighting Ebola, the affected countries cannot now care effectively and efficiently for other non-Ebola diseases.[200,201,243]

Lower GDP on health

As previously reported, prior to Ebola none of the West African countries met the required health GDP expenditures.[68] Thus, in view of the Ebola strike, it is to be expected that a far lower GDP will be allocated to health during the next couple of years in the most seriously affected countries.[57,244] One of the major problems facing the sub-regional countries is the lack of diversity in the economy. Therefore, when any portion of the economy falters, the remainder of the national economy may be expected to falter as well.[245] As one Liberian adage goes, "when someone pulls the rope, the rope will draw the bush, and everything in the bush will follow". Once Ebola triggered the spending spree on an already very meager health fund, the entire amount allocated for health became exhausted within a short period of time.

Reduced Physician-Patient ratio

More than 841 health workers in the sub-region contracted EVD. Of these, more than 500 died (see table 7). The fatality rate among the health workers that contracted Ebola was about 60%.[53] Prior to Ebola outbreaks in West Africa, the physician-patient ratio was about 1-2 per 100,000 people.[18, 53] Since so many health workers have died, that ratio is even worse, necessitating that each remaining doctor will have more patients to attend to.[58,255] The rate at which Ebola took the lives of the health workers was more than the pace necessary to train health workers to replace the fallen heroes and heroines. Furthermore, it would not seem strange should some of the health workers that survived Ebola fear to return to practice. Others may be expected to experience a post-Ebola syndrome or other form of post-Ebola disability that may compromise their capability.[256]

Table 7: Ebola and Health workers in West Africa

Country	Cases	Deaths	Fatality
Guinea	162	100	61.7%
Liberia	370	178	48.1%
Mali	2	2	100%
Nigeria	11	5	45.5%
Senegal	0	0	0%
Sierra Leone	296	220	74.3%
Total	**841**	**505**	**60%**

Health workers[53,96]

Orphans

At times the speed with which Ebola killed was so great that there was no time for the sick person to plan for caring for family members that were being left behind. According to UNICEF, there are over 10,000 Ebola-linked orphans in the West Africa sub-region.[257] Most of these orphans also suffer stigmatization and neglect.[258, 259] Since in many cases the children had been around their Ebola infected family members, relatives were often afraid to take them into their homes.[260]

Reduced orthodox health patronage

The message that there was no cure for Ebola was viewed by some in the sub-region as a failure of modern medicine and, therefore, a hopeless situation. As a direct result of the message some people would not go to the hospital for fear of contracting Ebola. As a result of the apparent failure of modern medicine, the rippling effects of Ebola caused a drastic reduction in the utilization of health services for other non-Ebola conditions in Freetown.[13,261] The post-natal clinic attendance when compared to that of 2013 was observed to be lower.[13]

More traditional health attendant patronage

There are many places in West Africa where accessibility, availability, and acceptability of modern medicine is still a big problem.[262] The reasons for this problem are rooted in such things as poverty, culture, neglect by the central government, and language barriers.[28] These are the same things that made the Ebola fight so difficult from the outset. In the most severely affected West African countries, the Ebola outbreaks were spreading in a centripetal-like fashion; that is, from the border towns with poor health facilities on the periphery towards the center (urban cities)[263] where there are centralized health care systems,[264] a high level of literacy, and information dissemination facilities such as radio, televisions, and billboards. There, too, the communication network tends to have better, clearer, and more regular services than those in the country sides.[265] These factors help in health education and prevention, especially in the cities and urban areas. Lacking these services in the villages and border towns,[88] the Ebola message that has to do with lack of cure and specific treatment tends to encourage people to continue to patronize the traditional health attendant.[266]

Reduced economy

The impact of Ebola outbreaks in West Africa can be seen in almost all facets of life.[11,13] The West African economy (including the three countries affected the most by Ebola) was growing rapidly even up to the first half of 2014, according to the World Bank update.[223] Unfortunately, largely because of Ebola, the projected 2014 national growth in Liberia was at 2.2% compared to 5.9% prior to the Ebola crisis and 2.5% in October 2014.[223] The projected 2014 national growth in Sierra Leone was at 4.0% (11.3% before the Ebola crisis and 8.0% in October 2014).[223] The projected 2014 national growth in Guinea was at trailing 0.5% (4.5% before the Ebola crisis and 2.4% in October 2014)".[223] According to UNDP, Guinea's government has a $220 million financing gap because of the Ebola crisis.[201] Ebola outbreaks led to a decrease in both demand (personal and household income, investment, and exportation) and supply (agricultural productivity and businesses), reduction in national growth, fall in budget revenue, increase in inflation, increase in public expenditure, and negative basic fiscal balance.[267]

Reduced workforce: The labor force in these most affected West African countries began to decline due to the death of the workers from Ebola, from Ebola panic/fear, flight of foreign expatriates, Ebola-induced disability, and government-directed closure.[267] In Liberia, about 60 percent of markets had been closed and about half of the mining and palm oil concessions had lowered their productivity and activity[11,13] Those that worked in the tourist industry soon noticed that tourists were no longer visiting for fear of Ebola, also resulting in job loss. Tourist guides, tourist bus-drivers, and antiquity sellers woke up to discover that Ebola had not only killed their relatives and devastated the nations they loved, but also killed their tourism jobs. Workers in the hotel industry realized that hotels once bubbling with foreign and local clients recorded drastically lower turnout.[267] They knew that without guests their jobs, too, were in danger of loss.[268] While the towns and major cities experienced about 50% work force loss, workforce loss in the rural areas was 75%.[267]

Working hour loss

Sickness: About 841 health workers contracted Ebola. Of these, 505 died.[53,96] The health sector lost the workers and the hours they could have invested if they had lived. Even those that lived could not return to work immediately after being tested and found to be free from Ebola.[96] Cumulatively, a sick worker might lose somewhere between 168 and 400 hours (or even more) to Ebola. And when there were many workers infected with Ebola, the health facility experienced shortage and over burdening of the available staff.

Quarantine: The incubation period of Ebola is 21 days, so the duration of the quarantine is the period of incubation of the Ebola virus.[1] A health worker quarantined for 21-days loses about 120-168 hours of working time. Because of this, a situation in which many health workers are quarantined, the health facility experiences a serious problem in providing full health services to the public.[96,269] The same thing is true in other sectors of society when staff members come in contact with the Ebola virus and must be quarantined for 21 days.[1] Individuals that are quarantined are expected to limit their interaction with the public in an effort to prevent spreading the Ebola virus should they subsequently be found to be infected by the Ebola virus. During the period of quarantine, suspects are expected to monitor their temperature and to report any elevation above 100.4°F (38°C) to the hospital without further delay.[1,2]

Isolation: The numbers of hours spent in isolation are dependent upon the health condition of the patient, severity of disease, and response to treatment. Staff members found to be positive to Ebola virus are isolated in order to properly treat and closely monitor the individual as well as to ensure that they are not transmitting the disease to others.[1,2] Those providing care to the isolated patients are fully gowned from head to toe.[1,2] Many hours are thus lost to the rigorous process of putting on the PPE and taking off the PPE. The range of hour's lost to isolation can range from 168 to 400 or more, depending on the severity of EVD, the pre-exposure immune status, nutritional status, treatment-response, and co-morbidity.[1,2]

Disability: This is very hard to quantify depending on the level of disability.[256] Those with permanent disability may not return again, while those with limited disability may return to work with accommodation when able.[256,270] The Ebola-induced disability results in a very significant loss to the workforce and national economy.[271,272]

Ebola myth

The Ebola myth cuts across all facets of life in the West Africa sub-region and beyond.[273] When Ebola first appeared no one really knew what it was all about, necessitating sometimes untrained substitutes to fill in the gaps.[274] Initially, even the health workers failed to diagnose Ebola because it was more of a new phenomenon than a specific disease to them.[275] Therefore, it took some time before it dawned upon health professionals that this was not just the usual case of malaria, shigellosis, or typhoid.[275] By the time people woke up to the reality of Ebola, many lives, dear lives, professional lives, children, women, bread winners, and others had been lost with no means of bring them back again.²⁷⁶ It was a real, colossal myth! It was not only the virulence or the degree of devastation and fatality that constituted the Ebola mythology, but the fear, scare, and panic that came with the inability to find an Ebola-specific therapy or timely cure.²⁷⁷ The spectrum of Ebola mythology includes transmission, complications, and the various folk-medicine remedies (eating raw onion, drinking high salt solution, and chewing bitter kola nut).²⁷⁸ Ebola might be eradicated in due course but the myth will linger for a while.

Social Stigmatization

In general, West African people are very loving, hospitable, and kind. In African culture people care for each other.²¹ However, fear of contracting Ebola is changing the hospitality and the caring attributes of the West African people. Because many of the people do not have a correct understanding of the post-treatment Ebola status, even those that have been treated for Ebola and declared free are not readily accepted back into society without some level of reluctance and hesitation...²⁵⁹ Unfortunately, this stigmatization extended beyond the primary Ebola victims. Their families and children were being discriminated against as well.²⁷⁹ Worse yet, orphaned children left behind by the Ebola-related deaths, were rejected and unwanted even by parents and relatives for fear of contracting disease from the children.²⁵⁹ In some communities, survivors are considered to be "witches" by people that view Ebola as a curse on those that practice witchcraft.²⁵⁶

Post-Ebola syndrome

The life of survivors undergoing isolation because of Ebola has sometimes been most devastating. Some came home to empty houses due to the death of other members of their families that were not as fortunate to have survived Ebola as they.²⁵⁶ Dr. Margaret Nanyonga, the WHO psychosocial support officer, observed that some of the Ebola survivors were complaining of problems with such things as clouded vision and gradual vision loss.²⁵⁶ Two Ebola survivors had actually become blind.²⁵⁶ She stated further that other problems seen in the post-Ebola syndrome also include body aches (joint, muscle, and chest pain), headaches, and extreme fatigue.²⁵⁶,²⁸¹ This syndrome impairs not only their activities of daily living, but in addition, their reintegration into the society and the ability to secure dependable jobs.[256,281] This post-Ebola syndrome can also predispose to a permanent disability.[256] In response to the great need, post-Ebola follow up consists of instructions to the survivors regarding how to deal with physical, psycho-social, economic, and Ebola-related post-traumatic stress.[256,280]

Possible short-lived Ebola surveillance

One of the major problems in West Africa is lack of maintenance and continuity.[281] Many times, lofty programs are begun that after a while disappear as into "thin air." We can learn from the experience with Ebola in East Africa how it occurs in an "off and on" fashion.[1] Therefore, discontinuing surveillance prematurely may make it impossible to detect a re-emergence of Ebola should it occur.[283] Likewise, we can apply the same approach to surveillance of other communicable diseases as we now have at the ports of entry and exit.[284]

Ebola-free declaration's milestone

Senegal

On August 20, 2014 a 21-year old Guinean arrived at a relative's home at the outskirts of Dakar.[285] He later developed fever, diarrhea, and vomiting symptoms which caused him to seek medical attention. He was treated for malaria as an out-patient on August 23, 2014.[285] Travel history was not known and he was not feeling any better. He was later admitted on August 26, 2014 at the specialized infectious disease center to which he was referred.[285] An alert from Conakry, Guinea, about a person that had escaped from the surveillance system and had had an earlier close contact with a confirmed Ebola patient, increased the Ebola high index of suspicion in his case.[285] Thus, he was investigated for Ebola and was confirmed to have the disease and this led to a cascade of contact tracing networking.[285]

The ministry of health, health workers, and the WHO's senior epidemiologists swung into actions that led to contact-tracing of 74 individuals that had had close contacts with the index patient.[285] Their temperatures were monitored twice daily and they were asked to report any symptoms they might feel. Only five of them developed non-specific symptoms of malaise and flu-like.[285] They, were tested and had negative results. On September 18, 2014, eight days after the confirmation laboratory results of the index patient, a subsequent negative laboratory test, and rapid improvement, he was discharged. Forty two days later, on October 17, 2014, in the absence of any new confirmed cases, Senegal was declared an Ebola-free nation.[285,286] It was a great joy to the nation to be Ebola-free. This brought great relief from the Ebola-tension, fear, and panic. The question one might ask is, "what factors are responsible for" the success story of Senegal?"

The Health Minister of Senegal, Dr Coll-Seck, presents the success story of Senegal in the neatly packaged summary the WHO below:

- The country had structured and willing political leadership right on top.
- The Ebola early detection and response with a well detailed plan and a prompt action by the National Crisis Committee.
- The national ports of entry and exit including those by roads had stepped up surveillance program.
- Resources were rapidly mobilized from both domestic and international sources that propelled the strong preparatory and readiness plans thus undoubtedly convincing the donors of the seriousness of the nation in tackling the Ebola outbreak.
- WHO and other operational partners also lent their indispensable support.
- Ministry of health and Welfare created a massive nationwide public awareness campaigns that utilized media experts and local radio networks and thereby provided the necessary feedback for the Ministry to self-monitor the emergency actions in place.
- Multi-disciplinary cooperation and collaboration among the government parastatals along with partnership with community leaders and think-tank ensured the desired ends.
- Socioeconomic support (money, food) as incentives and psychological counselling were provided for the patients and

patient contacts thereby leading to compliance and cooperation between the heath community and them.
- Reorientation and reintegration support were provided for the recovered patients and societal fear was alleviated that these Ebola survivors posed no risk of Ebola transmission to anyone.[285]

Nigeria

The index patient was fortunately picked up from the International Airport in Lagos and was taken to the hospital on July 25, 2014.[287] The type of Ebola spread in Nigeria was centrifugal-like in fashion (beginning in an urban area and spreading out to rural areas).[287] It started from the center (urban city, Lagos) which was different from the three Ebola-ridden West African countries where spread was centripetal-like (from rural to urban areas).[1,2,287] In centripetal Ebola spread, it was already established before the outbreak was noticed. Fortunately, with centrifugal spread it could easily be detected before being fully established.[288] That was one of the reasons for the efficient, effective, and prompt Ebola containment the world saw in Nigeria, defying the expected outright and full-blown Ebola outbreak predictions.[289] Most of the urban areas and cities in West Africa enjoy unparalleled access to good roads, good communication and network services, numerous print and electronic media services, billboards, posters, potable water, effective sanitary services, modern schools, and structured town planning systems in contrast to the villages, rural, and border towns.[290] Because of good roads, good communication and network services, and structured town planning systems[291] contact tracing becomes very easy. The level of literacy is very high in urban areas and cities[291] so there is no need for translation or misunderstanding as often occurs in the villages. It becomes easier to follow simple hygienic and sanitary guidelines since people in the urban areas[292] understand the rationale behind the recommended practices while those dwelling in the country often do not. Disinfectants are readily available in the urban centers but may be lacking in the rural and border villages, thus contributing to the spread of Ebola.[293] Nigeria was also fortunate because of the dedication of the health personnel and the staff at the first Consultant Hospital in Lagos who put their lives at risk to save the entire nation of Nigeria.[131]. In addition, the Polio epidemiologic, surveillance, and preventive team instantly got involved in Ebola contact tracing. All hands were on desk, beginning with the Nigerian government--federal, state, local; airports, media, Nollywood, WHO--to the NGOs that worked tirelessly and vigorously to identify, contact, and trace those that might have come in contact with the index patient.[287,294] With expertise, pragmatism, and experience, in due course Nigeria was able to show-case a world-class example of the containment of Ebola.[287] Ebola screening takes place at the ports of entry and exit and in the schools as well [294] In West Africa setting, centrifugal Ebola outbreak is better than centripetal Ebola outbreak.[293] Even though, the urban areas are more populated than the countryside, the fact remains that factors that are very important to fight the disease outbreaks are more readily available in the urban areas.[293,294] These factors include easy contact tracing, comprehensible dissemination of information, reduced culture shock, technologically enhanced health message (billboards, posters, flyers, cell phone instant message, internet), equipped health facilities, good laboratory, good roads, functional isolation units, quarantine compliance, hygiene compliance, availability of disinfectants, and a high educational level.[287,295] These factors contributed greatly to the Ebola containment success story of Nigeria despite the fact that Lagos and Port Harcourt were heavily populated.[287] If the Ebola index case in Nigeria had started in the remote part of the country it could have claimed many lives and taken more time to eradicate because the villagers would likely have first consulted the traditional medicinal practitioner who probably would not have recognized the disease Ebola.[262,296] The traditional medicinal practitioner could have become the focus of infection transmission since emphasis on hygiene is to them of minimal importance--a very important factor in fighting Ebola.[126,69] The experience of Nigeria supports unequivocally that it is easier to contain a centrifugal Ebola outbreak than a centripetal one (see table 7). What happened in Nigeria also supports the fact that Firestone in Liberia was able to contain the Ebola cases in no time while it was impossible to do the same in the slum areas of Liberia.[297] In West Africa, the pattern of distribution of basic amenities is, the closer one is to the central government, capital city, or commercial city the more the quantity and the higher the quality of the basic social amenities to be utilized.[298] It follows the law of direct proportionality. The reverse is the case, the farther away someone is from the central government, capital, or commercial city, the less the quantity and the lower the quality of the basic social amenities to utilize.[28,298] It follows the law of inverse proportionality. This is the rationale behind the health disparity in West Africa.[299,300] Nigeria saw how horrible and terrible Ebola had been in the sister ECOWAS countries of Guinea, Liberia, and Sierra Leone. There could be no excuse for her to say she had never heard about Ebola before. Learning from the experience of Ebola in Liberia, all hands were on desk to fight the Ebola war that was imported to Nigeria from Liberia. On October 20, 2014, Nigeria was declared Ebola-free by the WHO.[287]

Mali

On October 23, 2014, the first Ebola case in Mali was diagnosed in a 2-year old girl that was suspected to have lost about five of her immediate and extended families to Ebola in Guinea.[301] She was brought to Mali by her grandaunt. She was admitted to the hospital where she tested positive for Ebola, dying in the hospital on October 24, 2014.[301,302] Contact tracing was instituted and about 108 individuals were identified to have come in contact with the index case. Of these, 33 were health-care workers.[301] With the arrival of this case of Ebola in Mali, the former United States National Institutes of Health funded and well-functioning Biosafety level 3 laboratory for tuberculosis bacteria and HIV was repurposed for Ebola investigation and diagnosis.[301] On October 25, 2014 a Grand Imam from Guinea was admitted in Bamako, Mali for kidney failure and later died on the third day.[301-303] This case served as an Ebola virus seeding point. As a result of it, seven cases of Ebola were identified, of which five died, including a doctor and a nurse that had treated the Grand Imam.[301] In all, 433 contacts were identified and followed up for the 21-day incubation period of Ebola.[301-303]

In November 2014, Dr. Margaret Chan, WHO Director-General, visited an Ebola treatment center in Bamako, Mali she met with President Ibrahim Boubacar Keïta, Prime Minister Moussa Mara, and other government leaders in order to discuss strategies on tackling Ebola outbreaks in Mali and to show unflinching support by the United Nations.[304] On January 18, 2015 after 42 days of the last diagnosed case of Ebola in Mali, Mali was declared an Ebola-free nation.[305] Mali's success story emanated from the high level of vigilance that was crucial to the rapid detection of the first imported Ebola case and the commitment and involvement of the government, international community, and WHO epidemiologists.[301-303] It is pertinent to mention that Mali made all of her resources available to fight the Ebola war. This included the making of a national emergency declaration of Ebola, the use of medical students with training in epidemiology, emergency operations centers, and the use of an innovative telephone hotline to allay public fears and dispel public misconceptions, and rigorous and effective contact tracing.[301]

Possible vaccine

On October 23, 2014 the WHO convened a high-level emergency meeting at which more than 90 participants from around the world were in attendance to discuss Ebola vaccines, access, and financing.[306] The following resolutions[306] were reached:

- Impact of vaccines on further evolution of the epidemic
- Financing of vaccine development, clinical trials, and vaccination campaigns
- Liability
- The timing and quantity of vaccine supplies
- Design of protocols for phase 2 and phase 3 clinical trials
- Priority uses of vaccine when supplies are limited
- Regulatory requirements
- Urgent measures to improve readiness for clinical trials and vaccines
- Coordination and alignment among multiple partners
- Determination to finish the job

Table 8: Potential Ebola Vaccines

Vaccine / Company	Drug's mode of action	Vaccine against Ebola species	Available preclinical testing data	Available safety data	Remarks
cAd3-EBO; NIAID/ GSK vaccine	Induces a T-cell response, CD8 T cells production, immune protection against Ebola viruses.	Sudan and Zaire Ebola	Development of antibody and T-cell responses, and were sufficient to protect vaccinated animals from Ebola disease	No serious adverse events; high dose produced a brief sustained fever with the day of vaccination	Phase I Clinical trials; Single intramuscular (IM) injections at two dose levels.

VSV-EBOV; Public Health Agency of Canada, Merck, Wellcome Trust	Induces immune response against real Ebola virus	Zaire Ebola	Protective immune response in nonhuman primate (NHP)	No vaccination-induced fever or symptoms	A single IM dose
Advac / MVA-BN; Johnson & Johnson/ Bavarian Nordic	Combination of prime-boost regimen; one vector primes and another boosts immune response	Zaire Ebola	Protective immune response in NHP and relatively safe as well	Safe so far	Combo regimen
EBOV GP; Novavax Inc	Recombinant DNA that enhances immune response	.Zaire Ebola	NHPs were protected against EVD after being given the vaccine	No reported serious adverse vents	
University of Texas/ Austin	Breathable vaccine builds immune response against EVD	Zaire Ebola	Protective in NHP	Not yet tested in humans	Nasal spray
Vaxart's respiratory syncytial virus (RSV) tablet vaccine candidate; Vaxart Inc.	Rapid Immune response inducer	.Ebola virus	Not available	Hoping to start test in human	Tablet

Sources[307-313]

Possible therapeutics

Table 9 below is the WHO list of possible Ebola therapeutic categories, "summarizing the data on drugs that are either being tested or considered for testing in patients with Ebola virus disease (EVD), have already been used in patients with EVD, or which had been considered, but have been deemed to be inappropriate for further investigation."[314] Apart from those in Table 9 are other drugs that have been tried as possible therapeutics for Ebola. These include the antimalarial (Chloroquine), antibiotics (Erythromycin), anti-infertility (Clomid (Clomiphene)), antiviral (Interferon), antiviral (Interferon/Ribavirin), AVI-7537, and FX06.[314]

Table 9: Possible drugs for patients with EVD

Medication	Mechanism of Action	Animal model data	Drug safety	Other feasibility considerations
Brincidofovir	dsDNA viruses small molecules antiviral inhibitor. Theoretically may not work in Ebola that is RNA virus	NHP: PK profile feasibility problem. Guinea pig: PK and efficacy study underway. Mice: No efficacious benefits	Elevated Liver enzymes	Oral drug. Dosage: Twice weekly
Zmapp	Three monoclonal antibodies cocktail and produced in tobacco plants.	NHP: Recorded 100% survival, 5 days after virus infection.	Yet to establish safety study in humans	Possibly 15 treatment courses every 6 weeks.
TKM-100802	Ebola RNA cleaving small inhibitory RNA. Ebola strain sequence-specific.	NHP: 67-100% efficacy	Phase I safety study. Side effects: Chest tightness dizziness, tachycardia.	IV infusion. Requires refrigeration.
Zmab	Three monoclonal antibodies (mAb) cocktail.	NHP: 100% efficacy.	Yet to conduct human safety studies	For research purpose.

BCX-4430	Direct-acting nucleoside analogue.	NHP: 30-120 minutes post Ebola infection efficacy. Not efficacious at 48–72 hours. Mice: 100% protection against Ebola.	Phase I safety trial in progress.	Routes: Intramuscular (IM) or IV.
Zmapp from CHO cells	Three MAb cocktail. Glycosylation.	NHP: Studies underway	Human safety: Yet to be demonstrated	Research
Erlotinib / sunitinib	Anti-neoplastic agents	NHP: No known data yet Mice: 10/10 (IP route) in combination only.	Short-term use tolerability.	Very expensive
Favipiravir	Viral RNA-dependent RNA polymerase inhibitor. Antiviral RNA small molecules. Had Japanese approval for novel/pandemic influenza treatment.	Mice: protected at 300mg/kg. Nonhuman primate (NHP): antiviral effect seen; 2 log reduction in viraemia.	Tested in volunteers with 3.6g on first day followed then 800mg twice daily (BID). Unidentified safety issues Possible safety issue in hepatic pathology	Dosage: 200mg tablets; 6g/ first day Total drug required 30 tablets. Swallowing difficulty.
rNAPc2	Recombinant protein, anti-coagulant / anti-inflammatory	NHP: 33% Survival rate.	Thrombosis prevention demonstrated in in Phase I and Phase II trials.	Limited availability.

Potential medications[314]

Possible Mutations

Within the first month of Ebola outbreaks in West Africa, the Ebola virus had amassed 50 mutations.[315] Scientists using genetic sequencing are tracking the genetic constitution of the Ebola virus. By this they are monitoring the observed mutations to determine if they may be modifying its rate of adaptability and infectiousness.[315] It may be possible for the mutation to make it less lethal but more contagious.[315,316] So far the mutations seen in the Ebola virus have not increased the deadliness, adaptability, or contagiousness.[315,316] Ebola is a RNA virus just as HIV and influenza. This RNA property confers high rate of mutations.[316] Another concern is the possibility that a mutation may change its mode of transmission from direct contact with infected blood to becoming airborne.[316] Fortunately there is no observable evidence among other hematogenous (blood-borne) infections such as HIV and Hepatitis B virus of change from hematogenous spread to becoming airborne. Therefore it is expected that Ebola will follow the example of these blood-borne diseases that have not mutated their mode of transmission.[316]

Chapter Seven
Ebola multifactorial prognostic measures

A number of factors are responsible for the various outcomes of the Ebola outbreak in West Africa in terms of morbidity and mortality. These factors include the immune status of the people,[317] the level of preparedness,[318] the quality of the health facility equipment,[319] a high-level laboratory,[320] expertise of health personnel management,[321] and socio-economic status.[322] According to the Huffington Post, "Peter Piot, the director of the London School of Hygiene and Tropical Medicine, had stated that worsening conditions in West Africa contribute to a "perfect storm," including a growing population, decades of civil war, widespread government corruption, dysfunctional health systems and a growing distrust in Western medicine."[146] See pages 10 and 11

Table 10: Ebola pattern of transmission and outbreak-type-prognostic factors

Centrifugal Ebola Outbreaks	Centripetal Ebola Outbreaks
Started in the urban areas	Started in the rural areas/ slum
Heavily populated	Sparsely populated
Low bat contact chance	High bat contact chance
Low dependence on bush meat	High dependence on bush meat
High level of education	Low level of education
Good hygienic practice	Poor hygienic practice
Good health facility accessibility	Poor health facility accessibility
Good nutrition	Poor nutrition
Good medical compliance index	Poor medical compliance index
Good media coverage	Poor media coverage
Good disseminated information use	Poor disseminated information use
More likely to consult medical personnel	More likely to consult traditional healer
High level of health-need consciousness	Low level of health-need consciousness

Better roads	Worse roads
Good contact tracing	Poor contact tracing
High disinfectant availability	Low disinfectant availability
Flexible cultural practice	Rigid cultural practice
High economic status	Low economic status
Low mortality rate	High mortality rate
Seek for medical treatment early	Delayed in seeking for medical treatment
Prompt diagnosis	Delayed diagnosis
Good immune status	Poor immune status
Good communication/ network services	Poor communication/ network services
Good social amenities	Poor social amenities
Regular medical check up	Irregular medical check up
Greater physician-patient ratio	Lower physician-patient ratio
Good prognosis	Poor prognosis

Sources[1,2,7,11,13,16,183,256,317-320]

Table 11: General Ebola Eradication Prognostic factor

Positive	Negative
Multi-disciplinary collaboration	Unilateral effort
International involvement	No international involvement
High-quality laboratory	Poor quality laboratory
Strong political will power and policy	Weak political motivation
Early detection and response	Late detection and response
Socio-economic support for patient/family	Lack of socio-economic support
Durable surveillance system	Poor surveillance system
Multi-national cooperation	Lack of cooperation
Social re-integration and rehabilitation	Poor re-integration and rehab program

Classic Ebola awareness program	Poor Ebola awareness publicity
NGO, charity organizations involvement	No involvement
Conscientious de-stigmatization efforts	Stigmatization
Availability of Ebola-expert staff	Shortage of Ebola-expert
Ebola well-equipped health facility	Lack of Ebola well-equipped center
De-centralized health facilities	Centralized health facilities
Long-term Media involvement	Short-term media involvement
Good compliance with preventive measures	Poor or Non-compliance with preventive measures
Good isolation facilities	Poorly run isolation facilities
High level of preparedness	Poor preparation
National Ebola emergency declaration	No national emergency declaration
Port of entry and exit screening	Lack of screening
High use of technology: Cellphone	No technology use
Multi-factorial interventional approaches	Unilateral intervention
High GDP-health expenditures	Low GDP-health expenditures
Community cooperation	Apathetic and distrusted community

Sources[1,2,7,15,16,256,284,298,317-320]

Chapter Eight
Ethical issues in using unregistered interventions for EVD

Despite the fact that Ebola was first discovered in 1976, there is still no Ebola-specific treatment or vaccine. The current treatment for Ebola as noted above is symptomatic, supportive, and palliative in nature.[16] As noted also, the current Ebola outbreak in West Africa is unprecedented in morbidity and mortality.[1] Even though there are no FDA-approved therapeutics, there have been cases where yet-to-be-clinically tested drugs have been used for Ebola cases.[323]

Ethical Dilemmas in Ebola outbreaks

The ethical questions of these uses will follow:

Was it ethical to use unregistered interventions for EVD?

Was it ethical to have first used the unregistered interventions for the few patients with EVD in the US and not in West Africa with many patients with EVD?

Was it ethical for drug companies to fail to have developed interventions for EVD since Ebola was first discovered in 1976?

Ethics and Interventions

Historical accounts of ethics in research

Ethics, simply put, is the basis of the moral conduct of acceptable and unacceptable behavior in a society.[324] Unfortunately, it has often taken a scandal to awaken the consciousness of society to uphold ethical standards whenever there is an ethical deviation.[325] According to David Resnik's research ethics timeline, between 1932 and 2014 there were about 110 ethical related events in medical research.[324] Most of these were violations of/or deviations from the ethical fundamental rights such as a lack of respect of human dignity, a denial of autonomy, and injustice.[326,327] For example, the Tuskegee Syphilis study that was sponsored by the U.S. Department of Health enrolled 600 African Americans without study disclosure or obtaining informed consent for treatment for syphilis (Penicillin became available in mid-1940's). This in spite of the fact that the study design even included death as one of the outcomes.[328] The study started in 1932 and lasted through 1972 at which time public outcry against it led to its termination.[328] In May 16, 1997, President Bill Clinton officially apologized to the survivors and the families of all those that were used as subjects in the Tuskegee Syphilis study.[329] He said, "The United States government did something that was wrong -- deeply, profoundly, morally wrong. It was an outrage to our commitment to integrity and equality for all our citizens."[329] He further added, "The American people are sorry -- for the loss, for the years of hurt. You did nothing wrong, but you were grievously wronged.[329] I apologize and I am sorry that this apology has been so long in coming".[329]

Other examples of remarkable scandals include the Nazi's experiments and the Nuremberg trial in 1946-1947; the U.S. Public Health Service sexually transmitted diseases inoculation study in Guatemala, South America in 1946-1948; The Pfizer Trovan study in Nigeria in 1996; and Jessie Gelsinger human gene therapy experiment at the University of Pennsylvania, to mention just a few.[324, 328]

Fundamental ethical principles

The Belmont Report centered on ethical principles and guidelines for research involving human subjects: It distinguished the boundaries between practice and research, defined basic ethical principles, and applications of these principles in research.[330] According to the Belmont Report, the concept of practice connotes "interventions that are designed solely to enhance the well-being of an individual patient or client and that have a reasonable expectation of success" through diagnosis, preventive measures or therapeutics.[330] The term, research, refers to "an activity designed study to test a hypothesis, permit conclusions to be drawn, and thereby to develop or contribute to generalizable knowledge (expressed, for example, in theories, principles, and statements of relationships)" through a formal protocol that contains the study design, statistical analysis plan, data management plan, methods, and resulting interpretations.[330] The three basic ethical principles are respect for person, beneficence, and justice while the applications are informed consent, assessment of risk and benefits, and selection of subjects.[327,330]

Argument for ethical issues in using unregistered interventions for EVD in West Africa

Ethical rationale argument

It was ethical to use unregistered interventions for EVD.

There were no Ebola-specific therapeutics and the conventional care that was applied had not changed the high severity, mortality, and fatality rate of the disease.[331] Conventional care of Ebola at the time included supportive symptomatic care, palliation, psychosocial support, and nutritional support.[16] Therefore, it would have been unethical to just fold one's arms without trying to do something against the outbreaks.

It was ethical to have first used the unregistered interventions for the few patients with EVD in the US and not in West Africa with many patients with EVD.

The U.S. is well equipped with good health facilities having the capability to monitor any potential or idiosyncratic adverse drug events in preference to developing countries like Liberia, Guinea, and Sierra Leone that have no comparable means.[332] There are many infectious disease and emergency care experts in the U.S. capable of rapidly detecting and treating serious side effects that might arise from the use of unregistered interventions.[333] Compared to West Africa where it would be difficult because of language barriers to obtain full, comprehensive, informed consent, the same problem would not exist in the U.S.[334,335]

It was ethical for drug companies to have failed to develop interventions for EVD since Ebola was first discovered in 1976

The usual cost of first bringing a therapeutic concept to the bench, of doing pre-clinical studies, of clinical trials, and of finally bringing the agent to the bedside is about 5 billion dollars.[336] Since about 95% of experimental interventions fail in safety and efficacy when applied to humans, the cost of creating an effective agent would be practically prohibitive.[336] In view of the limited number of Ebola cases in the past, It would be difficult for any drug company to justify such expensive research.[337] Investing in so few previous Ebola cases would have made it difficult for a pharmaceutical company to recoup their investment--even resulting in the company declaring bankruptcy and thereby making it impossible for them to invest in research and development of therapeutics for diseases having a much greater incidence of occurrence.[338] By remaining in business, drug companies are contributing to advancement in science, increasing quality and quantity of patients' life, and sustaining the economy.[339]

Relevant facts

Supportive laboratory and animal testing results: Recently, laboratory tests utilizing animals (primarily non-human primates) to identify preventive and therapeutic measures against Ebola are promising, further reducing the need and ethical acceptability to consider the use of unregistered interventions for EVD.[340] According to the FDA, pre-clinical results are very important for clinical studies.[341] Therefore, if laboratory studies and animal testing were irrelevant to human studies, the FDA (the regulatory body) would not have made that as a necessary prerequisite for therapeutic trials in humans.[341]

High Ebola morbidity: As of March 29, 2015, the total number of cases (suspected, probable, and confirmed) of Ebola was 25213. Of these, 14347 were laboratory-confirmed.[342]

High Ebola mortality: The Ebola outbreaks in West Africa have been unprecedented in the history of this disease. Between the dates of March 25, 2014 and March 29, 2015, 10460 Ebola related deaths were recorded [342] With these alarming figures, it simply connotes that conventional care is not the best treatment choice and that having alternative interventions available even though still unregistered may be the most ethical choice.[101]

High Ebola fatality rate: The current fatality rate of EVD is around 50%. If nothing further is done to curtail the disease, the incidence and fatality rate may increase even farther.[342] Since conventional care is not scaling down the fatality rate, the use of an alternative with at least some therapeutic potential may be better that a placebo or of conventional care.[101]

High mortality of health workers: During the Ebola crisis, more than 841 health workers contracted EVD. 505 of these died of their disease--a fatality rate of 60%. [53, 96] Without a tangible approach to Ebola, we will not only continue to lose the lives of health workers.[343] Furthermore, others will be discouraged from entering the health-care world as well. It is therefore ethically acceptable and justifiable to have used unregistered interventions in order to build confidence and trust in the health community, and to safeguard their lives.[344]

Overwhelmed health facilities: Compromised by conventional care, the under-funded health facilities of West Africa were quickly overwhelmed by Ebola..[345] Since the conventional care had been overwhelmed, it was ethically acceptable to try other measures such as the unregistered drugs and vaccines.

Resolution effects

Ebola containment: Since conventional care did not contain the Ebola outbreaks, unregistered interventions were indicated on a trial basis.

There is a very real possibility that the Ebola virus could become a bioterrorist weapon, and if it were, and if unregistered interventions were available to help to contain the spread, it would be ethically justified, if not an ethical imperative to use them.[346] We are living in an age of terrorism. Terrorists are very desperate to lay their hands on whatever has the ability to cause catastrophic damage, inflict widespread pain, panic, and loss of life. In an effort to prevent such a terrorist event, prompt containment of this disease will deny their access to it.[347]

Improve quality of health life: Even though, it is too early to conclude, the majority of those treated with the unregistered interventions seem to have an improved quality of life when compared to those survivors of Ebola that were managed by conventional measures.[348] Many of those on conventional care later complained of symptoms now described as the post-Ebola syndrome--a condition that presents with body aches (joint, muscle, and chest pain), headaches, visual difficulty, and extreme fatigue[256]

Prolong quantity of life: The majority of those that were treated with the unregistered interventions have not died from the disease.[349] They continue to be monitored for possible side effects of the interventions.

Compassionate use: It is also called "expanded access" that allow patients with serious diseases or conditions to have access to investigational interventions.[350,351] This "compassionate use pathway" provides the "most to gain or the least to lose" patients with the interventional opportunity of investigational drugs, medical devices, or biologics.[350,352] Ebola is a very serious disease, so under the compassionate use act, it is ethically permissible and acceptable to use unregistered interventions.[353]

Relevant ethical considerations

Respect for the person: This is one of the cardinals of Belmont Report's ethical principles.

Autonomy: The decision to use unregistered interventions should rest solely on a competent adult with capacity to make a decision.[354] Every competent adult should be allowed to exercise their autonomy. When a competent adult is denied the choice to use an unregistered intervention, it is a constitutional rights infringement.[355]

Informed consent: It is a voluntarily signed document authorizing that the recipient of a proposed therapy or intervention has been fully informed regarding potential risks and benefits. When applied to the use of an unregistered intervention the individual also acknowledges that he/she understands that the unregistered intervention may have possible serious life-threatening complications, including death,[356] that he/she is consenting voluntarily without being coerced, and is taking responsibility for the actions by way of signature or figure printing.[357] The individual retains the right to withdraw the consent at any time without being penalized for doing so.[358] A competent adult can sign an informed consent and a legal representative of a minor can sign and the minor at certain age can assent as well.[359] A legal custodian may sign informed consent for an incompetent individual.[359]

Privacy and confidentiality: For the fact that an individual consenting to the use of an unregistered intervention may be ill with Ebola does not negate the rights to privacy and confidentiality of their health information.[360]

Preservation of dignity: The individual receiving unregistered interventions must be treated with all due respect without losing their dignity.[340] The unregistered interventions should not diminish any one's right to human dignity. Everyone must be properly cared for and be given the best possible available care.

Beneficence: In giving unregistered interventions, one must ensure that one does not commit any harm.[360] Preventable harm should be averted as much as possible.

Preclinical reports: Data generated from pre-clinical studies of these interventions should be properly studied before the use of these interventions on humans.

Laboratory findings: The laboratory findings showed some favorably promising results. These are results from animal testing and cell studies.[340]

Animal testing: According to the August 11, 2014 report of the WHO advisory panel on ethical considerations for use of unregistered interventions for Ebola viral disease, one of the pivotal reasons for supporting the use of unregistered interventions was the fact that laboratory and animal models' gave promising results of these interventions.[340] Especially in non-human primates, these interventions demonstrated efficacy, potency, and safety.[340] According to an FDA investigational new drug requirement, laboratory and animals data are very important factors to be considered prior to the commencement of clinical trials.[341]

Risk-benefit assessment: Ethical soundness demands scientific integrity and benefit that outweighs risk.[327, 361,362] In using unregistered interventions in Ebola patients, one extrapolates from the pre-clinical findings that have already shown benefit over risk.[340] Based on these pre-clinical findings, it is expected that the unregistered interventions will potentially benefit human.[340] This supports the ethical rationale for the use of unregistered interventions in patients with Ebola.

Justice: Having ethically considered the acceptable facts under which unregistered interventions can be used, [340] the questions remaining to be answered on the limited numbers of interventions are: Who gets the unregistered interventions? What criteria should one use in the distribution of the unregistered interventions?

Distributive justice: There should be fairness in the distribution of the unregistered interventions between countries with Ebola disease and among the Ebola-stricken population within a country.[340] In social justice and fairness, the benefits and the burdens of the unregistered interventions should be equitably distributed.[363]

Social usefulness: Some believe that since health care workers are so essential to society for the management and containment of Ebola they should be socially prioritized in the distribution of unregistered interventions.[340, 364] They should be first to receive the limited supply of unregistered interventions with the intent that they would recover more rapidly and return to their post of helping the ill as quickly as possible. Some would also argue for the motivational effect produced by priority access to unapproved drugs or vaccines in encouraging others to enter the healing professions.[365]

Reciprocity: Those that favor prioritizing health personnel in the distribution of yet-to-be approved interventions bring to the table the law of reciprocity. Applications of the law of reciprocity demand that because health workers put their lives on the line to help society, so it is time for the society to place them first in line for the distribution of the unregistered interventions.[340] Protagonists contend that "the same argument should hold for paramedics and the families of the health workers and the health-related work".[340]

Dr. Felix I. Ikuomola

Argument against ethical issues in using unregistered interventions for EVD in West Africa

Ethical disagreement

It was not ethical to use unregistered interventions for EVD

Insufficient information on the interventions: The information about the unregistered interventions are still relatively scanty. Therefore, using interventions with limited information regarding toxicity, safety, efficacy, and potency upon humans is unethical.[366] When we fail to learn from the history of past failures we are bound not only to repeat, but to perpetuate the vicious cycle of the past rather than promoting a virtuous cycle for the future.[328]

It was not ethical to have first used the unregistered interventions for the few patients with EVD in the US and not in West Africa with many patients with EVD.

More life-threatening outbreaks in West Africa: While there were thousands of people infected and dying of Ebola in West Africa, only four cases of Ebola were seen in the U.S.[2] Administration of unregistered interventions to the Ebola patients in the U.S. was ethically untenable and illogical since we have more patients suffering and dying from Ebola in West Africa than in the U.S.

Health disparity: Giving unregistered interventions to the American patients but not to the Ebola-stricken West African patients was clear evidence of health disparity[367,368] between the wealthy and the poor—and between the developed and the under-developed countries. There was no ethical logic in singling out patients in the U.S. for the unregistered interventions while thousands of non-U.S. patients with Ebola died of the disease in West Africa. Does this mean that one must be a U.S. citizen to be the first to receive unregistered interventions? Does it mean that if those patients in West Africa had been U.S. citizens that all of them would have been first-in-line to receive the unregistered intervention?

It was not ethical for drug companies to have failed to develop interventions for EVD since Ebola was first discovered in 1976

Profit-driven: The primary goal of pharmaceutical firms and biotechnology should not be profit-driven, but patient-driven.[369] When this basic principle of patient before profit is ignored, the pharmaceutical company and biotechnology are bound (naturally inclined) to compromise patient safety and welfare, drug efficacy and effectiveness, and professional ethics.[327] If pharmaceutical firms and biotechnology had done something about Ebola when it was first discovered in 1976, the Ebola outbreaks with unprecedented deaths in West Africa probably could have been averted. Many lives that were lost to the Ebola war would have been saved and the Ebola epidemic would have been contained. As the saying goes, "A stitch in time saves nine" but the pharma did not apply this simple maxim of life.

Orphan drug status: If the pharmaceutical companies and biotechnology had put patient before profit they would have applied the Orphan Drug Act of 1983 that was enacted to facilitate the discovery, development, and commercialization of interventions to manage rare diseases.[370] By applying the Orphan Drug Act, pharmaceutical companies or biotechnology would have been able to develop drugs and vaccines for Ebola and would have also avoided incurring financial loss. Ethically, socially, and legally, there is no justifiable reason for the drug companies not to have developed interventions for Ebola prior to this time of explosive Ebola outbreaks.

Interventions' efficacy unpredictability

From an evolutionary biologic point of view, one should expect species differences in anatomy (structures), physiology (functions), pharmacodynamics, pharmacokinetics (absorption, distribution, excretion, and metabolism), pharmaco-toxicity, and in the DNA repair mechanism.[371,372] In fact this has frequently been the case in pharmacological research. There have been drugs that have passed both efficacious and safety tests in animals, but failed in humans. For example, the sedative, Thalidomide, caused birth defects in human, [373] and the anti-arthritic, Vioxx, caused heart attacks and sudden cardiac death in humans.[374] Whereas, there have also been drugs that were unsafe and ineffective in animals, but have shown to be efficacious and safe in humans.

These include Aspirin, poisonous in cats; anti-transplant rejection Fk-506 (tacrolimus), unsafe in some animals, and penicillin, guinea pig toxicity.[375,376] Only about 5% of the drugs that work in animals pass the efficacy and safety testing in humans, and about 95% do not really predict how humans will respond.[375,377,378] There are some issues of publication bias that often overestimate the animal results.[379] Animal models do not actually resemble human internal milieu even in chimpanzees, 99%, and, mice, 98% with human genetic similarities, respectively.[380] In a statement Dr. Richard Klausner, former director of the National Cancer Institute (NCI), made to the Los Angeles Times, he said, "We have cured cancer in mice for decades—and it simply didn't work in humans".[376] Not everyone that contracted Ebola died from the disease, so how can we be sure that promising interventions in animals will make any difference? In considering this question, we must acknowledge that it would have been ethically prudent to have conducted thorough clinical trials before the use of these interventions in human. Based on the aforementioned facts, it was unethical to have based the use of unregistered interventions on humans from animal studies alone.

Possible severe adverse events

Adverse drug reactions in the U.S cost about 136 billion dollars annually.[381] Each year, adverse drug reactions account for about 20% of the injuries and deaths occurring among hospitalized patients.[382] When compared to controls, the mean hospital length of stay, costs, and mortality, for patients with adverse drug reactions are doubled.[383] In the case of Ebola, it would have been possible for the unregistered interventions to have had unanticipated adverse events which could have proven to be life-threatening, and even deadly, so there was no logical reason to allow unregistered intervention use in humans without prior clinical trials.

Ethical soundness versus ethical acceptability

The argument put forward by those in support of the use of unregistered interventions in humans was ethical acceptability.[340] Ethical soundness[384] and ethical acceptability are not totally the same and may not always be used interchangeability. They have ethical distinctiveness.[385] Ethical acceptability is at times anchored on emotional connotation[382,383] and social suitability.[383,386] It is possible for an issue to be ethically acceptable without being fully ethically sound. Whatever is ethically sound is almost always deemed to be ethically acceptable. More so ethical acceptability is relative. Ethical acceptability was the argument put forward by Nazi physicians[387] because it was ethically acceptable to them to conduct research on the victims whereas the rest of the world and the Nuremberg trial panelists believed that it had no ethical soundness.[388, 389] Ethical acceptability cannot trump ethical soundness. Ethical acceptability in this case was based on the fact that the Ebola outbreak was killing many people at a time when conventional care was doing nothing to halt or reduce the high level of mortality. However, there was no ethical soundness in the use of unregistered interventions for Ebola in spite of the ethical acceptability since these investigational interventions have neither undergone clinical trials to determine either efficacy and safety nor been approved by the regulatory authority such as FDA.

Discussion

We cannot deny the Ebola outbreaks in West Africa nor the unprecedented morbidity, mortality, fatality, and disability they has caused.[1, 2] We also know that the positive effects of conventional care seem not to be promising or containing the Ebola outbreaks.[390] We must just keep looking for something that will contain the outbreaks before we all become Ebola victims directly, or indirectly through bioterrorism. A greater fear is for Ebola to be used in bioterrorist war.[347] In order to utilize the promising laboratory and animal studies of unregistered interventions for potential benefits against Ebola virus in humans, ethical, scientific, and pragmatic considerations are very important.[340]

Application of Ethics

Ethical Committee of the institution: In order to make use of unregistered interventions it is important for the Ethics Committee of the institution to review and weight the benefit and the risk.[391] The involvement of the institutional ethics committee will help to ensure that ethical guiding principles are applied and complied with.[392] The role of the ethical committee is to ensure that patient dignity, safety, and wellbeing are protected, and that Clinician-Scientists put ethics before science as they conduct feasibility trials.[393]

Ethical criteria: Necessary ethical criteria including provision of special safeguards for the Ebola vulnerable groups such as children and pregnant women must be met in order to use unregistered interventions.[394] Since the unregistered interventions are still limited in supply, transparency and accountability are very germane to how these interventions are being distributed between nations and among human populations within the same countries.[340] In the course of the administration of these unregistered interventions, standard supportive and palliative care must be adequately and efficiently provided to the patients that are receiving the agents.[340]

Moral obligations: Those that are involved in the use of these unregistered interventions have moral obligations to adequately report any generated data for scientific and statistical analyses.[340] Interim analysis[395] of the data must be conducted for evaluation on the safety and efficacy of these unregistered interventions. If these interventions are not safe then it is the moral duty of the Clinician-Scientists or the researchers to terminate the use, and if these interventions are not better than the conventional care there is no need to continue its use as well.[396]

Appropriate consent process: West Africa is an underdeveloped sub-region. Therefore, in providing consent forms, the level of education, languages, and other specific needs must be considered.[397] Age-appropriate, education-appropriate, and language-appropriate consent forms need to be seriously considered in order for the people to comprehend[398] what the term, unregistered interventions, means. It must also be clear that they are not being forced to take the unregistered interventions. It is their inalienable rights to choose whether or not they wish to take them,[399] and to understand that they can withdraw their consent[400] at any time before the administration of the unregistered interventions.

Scientific integrity

Proper design: There is need to properly design these experimental interventions with provision for proper reporting and emergency management.[340] Necessary equipment for the use of these experimental interventions and monitoring for adverse events must be in place before the administration of these agents.[401]

Conduct: The protocol as approved by the institutional ethics committee must be followed, and if there is any deviation, approval from the same body should be sought.[402] These unregistered interventions must be stored according to the manufacturer's recommended temperature to ensure potency.[403] Failure to comply with the storage temperature may affect the efficacy, potency, and data generated from the unregistered interventions.[403] The monitoring plan should include quality assurance, control, and improvement.[404,405]

Proper reporting: The generated data need to be properly recorded and analyzed. These data must also include information regarding adverse events, with specific details on severity, types, duration, and alleviating and aggravating factors.[405]

Data validity: Transparency and ethical professionalism in data collection and extrapolation are very important.[340,406] Trust in, and patient safety, of these unregistered interventions hang on scientific integrity and data validity, so any data falsification and/or fabrication will compromise the statistical analysis.[407]

Data inference: The ultimate goal is to deduce inference from the data gathered during the use of the unregistered interventions in order to determine their efficacious superiority, non-inferiority, or bio-equivalence.[408] The data will also include safety issues, optimal dose, side effects, and some possible idiosyncrasy of these agents.[340]

Pragmatism

Health facility's standard: Quality health infrastructures should be in place in order to make use of unregistered interventions.[340] Functioning health infrastructures are needed for proper monitoring of the interventions.

Health personnel expert: Ebola is a serious, life-threatening, hemorrhagic disease.[409] There is need to have Ebola health experts on hand when the unregistered interventions are administered on patients so as to ensure maximum patient safety in case of any severe adverse events.[340,410]

Ebola-specific emergency training: There should be Ebola-specific emergency training[411] since infectious disease experts are limited. These efforts should be in place before the administration of the unregistered interventions to ensure patient safety and wellbeing and drug efficacy.[340]

Fast-track health facility upgrading/ capacity: Feasibility factor is a very important criterion before the administration of the unregistered interventions.[412] Without good facility feasibility it is impossible to apply good science and sound ethics.[413] Where the health facility is substandard there should be a fast-track upgrading.[414] There must be adequate capacity (hospital beds, equipment, materials, and logistics) in order to meet any eventuality that may arise from the use of the unregistered interventions.[340,413]

Double set-up

Trial-Care: Administration of unregistered interventions is a combination of simultaneous clinical trials and medical care.[340] The set up for data collection on safety, efficacy, adverse events, statistical analysis and reporting, imply clinical trials. Supportive care, counselling, treatment, or vaccination denotes medical care.[340, 414]

Bioethical Summary

Balancing ethics, science, and pragmatism: In using unregistered interventions for Ebola there is a need to strike an important balance in ethics, science, and pragmatism.[340] Ethics is vital to human dignity preservation, safety, and wellbeing.[415] Science is also important in drug discovery, development, and efficacy.[416] Without feasibility it will be difficult to administer the interventions. Human beings should never be means to the ends.[417] In the case of Ebola with alarming morbidity, mortality, and fatality, ethical acceptability should be considered along with the scientific integrity and pragmatism.[340]

Balancing Hippocratic Oath and reciprocity and social usefulness: It is true that the Hippocratic Oath demands unalloyed medical personnel responsibility to their patients first[418] while reciprocity and social usefulness put health personnel first in the distribution of limited unregistered interventions before their patients.[340, 413] The fact remains that patients need health personnel to attend to them, and not the other way round. So in order for the health personnel to be fit to attend to them they have to be alive to perform their professional duty.[340] In order for the health personnel to be alive to attend to patients they may need these unregistered interventions first.

Professional obligations: In gathering the data for the unregistered interventions transparency, trustworthiness, and scientific integrity should be uppermost.[340] The data should be thoroughly analyzed and inference made on whether these unregistered interventions are safe in human use with high quality drug efficacy or not.[340]

Chapter Nine
Prevention and Control of Ebola

The WHO and CDC have comprehensive Ebola guidelines that are very important in preventing and controlling the outbreaks. Below, these guidelines are divided into various units.

Public guidelines

- Community engagement with everyone participating and being considered as stakeholder.[419]
- Effective Ebola awareness communication in simple language, dialects, posters, billboards, dramatic arts, and media.[420]
- Good sanitation and hygiene practices.[421]
- Prompt and safe burial practices.[422]

Health workers/ Care givers guidelines

- Full body-covering-personal protective equipment (PPE) (face shield or goggles, long-sleeved gown and gloves, hoods, and booths) should be worn.[421, 423]
- Regular hand washing with disinfectant (0.5% Chlorine) solution and/or disinfectant lotion.[421, 423]
- Safe injection practices and safe burial practices.[423]
- Efficient case management, surveillance and contact tracing.[421, 424]
- Identification of people who may have been in contact with someone infected with Ebola for monitoring the health of contacts for 21 days.[423, 425]
- Quarantine and isolation as required in order to separate the healthy from the sick to prevent further spread.[423]
- Proper infection control and sterilization measures practices.[423]
- Always avoid direct, unprotected contact with the bodies of Ebola patients or corpses.[421, 423]
- If at any time one comes in contact with body fluids of an Ebola infected patients or corpse, one must notify the appropriate authority immediately.[423]

Laboratory Guidelines

- Good Laboratory practices compliance.[423]
- Only Ebola well-equipped laboratory should process the samples.[426]
- Blood, urine, saliva, and other samples from patients are an extreme biohazard risk, so maximum biological containment conditions are required.[423, 426,427]
- Samples from humans and animals should be handled with care.[423]

Animal guidelines

- Animals should be handled with gloves and other appropriate protective clothing.[2]
- Animal products (blood and meat) should be thoroughly cooked before consumption.[2]
- Routine cleaning and disinfection of monkey farms.[428]
- Quarantine the animals immediately if an outbreak is suspected.[429]
- Cull the infected animals with safe burial practices or cremation.[429, 430]
- Restrict or ban the movement of animals to avoid infecting other animals or human.[428,431]

Travel warnings

- Careful hygiene practice (Hand-washing with soap and water or an alcohol-based hand sanitizer.[423]
- Avoidance of coming in contact with blood and body fluids (clothes, bedding, needles, and medical equipment that might have been in contact with infected person).[421-423]
- Avoid coming in contact with an Ebola corpse during funeral or burial rituals.[421, 422]
- Avoid wild animal (bats and nonhuman primates) or their body fluids contact.[423, 428]
- Avoid Ebola treatment facilities in West Africa.[432]
- Do a 21-day self-monitoring after you return and seek medical care immediately if you developed symptoms of Ebola.[432]

Chapter Ten
Ebola-related Memories

This section was written by those who either treated Ebola, lost loved ones to Ebola, visited West Africa during the Ebola crisis, worked in the same place with the West Africa returnee, or had previously worked in Africa.

Storylines

Treating Ebola in Sierra Leone

Dr. David Koroma worked in Sierra Leone and treated many Ebola patients at his Ebola treatment center. He recounted horrors of Ebola and the frustrations he experienced from the cultural practices of the people that aided the spread of Ebola.

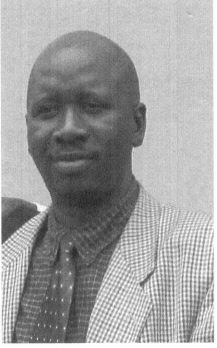

Fig.16: Dr David Koroma

At our Ebola center, it was mandatory for all the staff to undergo two to three weeks IPC (Infection Prevention Control) training. Our 66-bed capacity center was professionally staffed by two national doctors, 57 national nurses, 2 community health officers (CHO), 15 Cuban doctors, and 20 Cuban nurses. We also had a maternity wing for pregnant women with Ebola positive results.

We treated the first Ebola patient in our center on the 20th of December, 2014. We reopened the center on March 7, 2015 and had seen 191 patients, 32 of which had died.

Patient were either brought in by ambulance or self-reported at the Ebola center. They often presented with fever (38^{0}C), vomiting, redness of eyes, body pains, general body weakness, and diarrhea or rash.

Prior to patient admission to the Ebola center, we first triaged, screened and took blood sample for PCR testing. It usually took about 24 – 36hrs before we received the results. If the laboratory was very busy it took a longer time.

We isolated positively tested patients and advised them to use a commode bucket instead of the general toilet facility. They should not touch or be in contact with any other people until they had tested negative, at which time they would no longer be considered contagious. Basically, treatment was symptomatic, supportive, and provided along with counseling. We gave fluids for rehydration, antibiotics, and an immune-booster. When the patients were discharged, a lot of information was passed on to them on the dos and don'ts, especially on post-treatment sexual activities. They were advised to either abstain or to use condoms for 3 months from the time of discharge since some studies showed that semen and vaginal fluids of Ebola patients could remain infective for 3 months following successful treatment.

We also advised the families of the patients that until the patient tested negative they should not come in contact with them without PPE. The families were also counseled and encouraged to have hope that their patients could be among the Ebola survivors. We told them that when the patients were tested negative they were no longer able to transmit the disease and that the patients should be accepted back to the family and community.

There was an Ebola scare among the health personnel for fear of contacting Ebola from the Ebola center. Those that lost their friends and colleagues to Ebola felt the greatest fear. Work at Ebola center required a lot precaution. It was required that one must ensure that the PPE was put on before attending to any patient. The Ebola scare also gripped the people in the community where the Ebola center was located. Some could not understand why we allowed our hospital to be used as one of the Ebola centers in the country. However as time passed by the community came to terms with the reality of Ebola and acknowledged the service our center was rendering. Everyone, including the spiritual leaders of churches and mosques joined in a national season of prayer and fasting to fight the Ebola outbreaks despite the general belief that Ebola was a result of the evil practices of the people in the country. Ebola spread was perpetuated by traditional healers and traditional burials and rituals. The traditional healers did not practice safe hygiene while applying their medicinal. They had close contact with the patients without PPE.

It worth mentioning that the government played a significant role in controlling the epidemic through mass sensitization, posters, and media. The health information was centered on prevention and safe practices.

There were travel restrictions in order to facilitate Ebola containment. Other control measures included hand washing, safe burial practices, and prompt seeking behavior. Ebola brought economic depression, unemployment, starvation, social discrimination, and school closures. Ebola also led to an increase in numbers of deaths of widows and orphans.

Sweet Liberia

Trinida Kollie-Jones, RN, BSN, MSN (c), NP (c) hailed from Liberia and lost her childhood friends, husband, relatives, and neighbors to Ebola in Liberia. She gave the accounts in her own words, her heart-felt pain and disappointments.

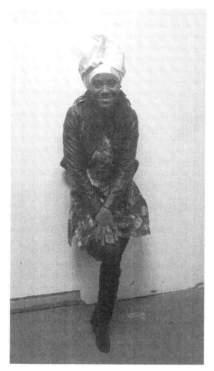

Fig .17: Trinida Kollie-Jones

The countdown continues as Liberians, as well as the rest of the world, keeps a close eye on Liberia to be declared Ebola free. I wonder how long it will take Liberia to be free of this Ebola virus. Has the process of entering Liberia via road been reviewed? How ready is the nation's healthcare system, infrastructure, etc., to deal with another Ebola outbreak or worse…. a disease that may require an airborne precaution if mutated to that level of severity? Has creating awareness, educating and providing training to the healthcare providers and the front lines been determined a vital component in keeping Ebola out of Liberia?

These are just a few of the many questions racing through my mind when I think about Ebola, how it has shaped my thinking, my country (Liberia), and the lives of many of my friends and even my family. Remembering the aroma, running up and down the halls, laughing as loud as I could in the yard are memories I try to hold on to when I think about my times as a child at the John F. Kennedy Memorial Hospital (JFK), one of Liberia's major government hospitals. Incredible and hardworking nurses made my times there the most peaceful, which played a major role in me becoming a nurse.

If only I could rewind the clock, I might be tempted to take it back to those days when I was a child; but I would not want that. Today, I am a wife, a mother to three beautiful children, and more importantly, I am a Registered Nurse. I, however, will not hesitate to rewind my clock to December of 2012, my last trip to Liberia. The smiles on the faces of my family, childhood friends, neighbors, and yes, some of those nurses that still work at JFK made me realize that many of our dreams had come to fruition, especially for three of my childhood friends. Two were registered nurses and one was a Physician Assistant. These are friends that at times, on many occasions, we would all sit out at night looking at the stars in the skies, discussing our dreams of becoming nurses and healthcare providers; how together we would contribute and have effective changes to the healthcare sector. We sang in the choir together at church. I was impressed with one in particular that I called a sister. We shared clothes, ate together and were considered by many as inseparable. She later became my sister-in-law and had a child by my brother. I remember and can picture how wide her smile was, from ear to ear when she explained to me how proud she was to have finally achieved her dreams and is now ready to begin living her life. She was now practicing as a Physician Assistant and living in her very own home, which she had built. She had a job she loved and she felt extremely satisfied.

During the Ebola outbreak she called me to inform me that Ebola had claimed the life of one of our friends. This friend was a nurse working at Phebe Hospital. We talked a lot about our loss and how her death impacted the church, the community and more importantly, her family. We laughed over the good times we shared singing in the choir. "Oh, you guys be very careful," I told her. Then we had the scare of our family trial times. I received the call at 2 am E.T. and never went back to sleep. My uncle, his children along with some of the other families were placed in quarantine for the next 21 days. His wife had fallen ill, and when she thought she was feeling worse instead of better after taking some Malaria medications, she checked herself into an Ebola unit and tested positive. My aunt-in-law died three days later but for the rest of the 21 days it was a nightmare I would not wish on anyone.

We Googled the CDC website and began educating our families and neighbors in Liberia on how they could prevent contracting this virus. Facebook became our go to information line, as every two minutes someone updated his or her profile that someone had died. We were eager to read it hoping that it was not one of our family members or friends. Then I got a call from my husband's sister that they had received a call that her husband's brother, along with his two step daughters had died from Ebola. From there on, it was one bad news after the other, from public figures, former beauty queen, neighbors, and so on. At this time, reality had hit home and I wondered to myself, wow, this is bad. But it got worse.

I will never forget the call I received that Saturday morning informing me that my childhood friend, sister and my brother's baby's mother, the Physician Assistant had come down to Monrovia with complaints of foot pain that Thursday, went to the hospital on Friday and had died on the Saturday of that same week. I was shocked and all I could think of was "*Oh Ebola.*" I was told that she had asked on that Friday to be checked for the Ebola Virus and that the preliminary results were negative. What else could it be? I was not thinking about myself at this time, all I thought about was the last sentence of this conversation, "We are depending on you to please find a way to inform her daughter about her death." This happened to be one of the most difficult things with which I have ever been entrusted. I felt broken, and at the same time angry at no one thing or person in particular, just very angry.

I took a closer look at the system, culture, education or lack of education (awareness), the infrastructure or lack of, area(s) of concentration of Liberia (population), and sanitation and I concluded that all are major contributors that aided the rapid spread of Ebola. Also, the health system, the government, that stigmatization that certain persons are better than others and are somehow not susceptible to a certain illness, especially those of high status, as well as the habit of most Liberian's to get their stories and information from many different places other than from the source. I would also say that the religious belief, as well as the family dynamics and Liberian way of doing things, such as shaking hands as a formal form of greeting or the willingness to help either friends, neighbors, or family members also help with the spread of Ebola.

I continue to carry that hope in my heart, that those plans we dreamt of all of those years ago of being contributing factors to Liberia's health system will continue to be fulfilled. Ebola is now gone from Liberia, but unforeseen consequences of its presence will hover over Liberia for years to come.

Trip to Nigeria

Dr Felix Ikuomola who had worked in many West African countries including Liberia and Sierra Leone before the Ebola epidemic traveled to Nigeria when Ebola was still raining horrors in the three badly affected West African states. He worked at Medway Hospital that was opposite the First Consultant Hospital in Lagos, Nigeria, where the Ebola index patient that brought the disease from Liberia to Nigeria was taken to. He had the time to discuss with friends and neighbors that were around when the index patient was brought to the hospital. He gave the vivid account of the reality of the Ebola disease, Ebola myth, and Ebola perspectives as related to him by the fellow Nigerians.

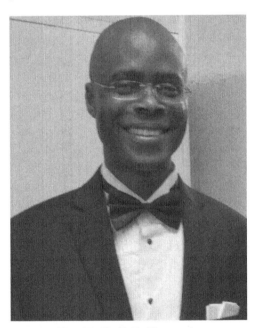

Fig. 18: Dr Felix Ikuomola

I went to Nigeria in December, 2014. As the plane was about to land at the Murtala Mohammed Airport, Lagos, Nigeria, an Ebola screening form was handed to everyone to be filled in. The questions ranged from which countries you have visited before coming to Nigeria, your country of departure, if you have come in contact with anyone sick with Ebola, or someone experiencing symptoms of Ebola such as fever and others. On arriving, we were scanned with a temperature reader before being allowed into the country. This was a new experience for me since I had never had anything like this before since I began traveling. Questions began to enter into mind. What if the temperature scanner did not accurately read the temperature? Could there be any factory failure in the calibration of the temperature scanner? Finally, I was happy, for the scanner showed that I had a normal temperature. I still continued to ponder on these questions as I waited for what seemed like forever for my luggage.

I used to work at Medway Hospital, Lagos before I began to travel. Medway Hospital is opposite the First Consultant Hospital, Lagos, where the Ebola index patient had been taken to. In the past I had visited First Consultant to see some of my colleagues with whom I had worked previously. Getting back to Nigeria I saw some of my old friends and noticed that nothing had really changed from the way it was before I left it many years ago. I was interested in hearing about the reactions of my friends and some other people about Ebola.

The majority of the people I talked to said they had never heard about Ebola before and did not even know what Ebola was all about until that Liberian man came to Nigeria. They said the news caught them unaware and most of them decided to bypass the main road of St. Gregory's college for a couples of weeks. They did not even come to Obalende bus-stop. I spoke to some Christian friends who believed that Ebola was one of the pestilences of the end time events the Bible talks about in Luke 21: 11, "There will be great earthquakes, famines and pestilences in various places, and fearful events and great signs from heaven."

Some people also told me how they were looking for possible preventive measures since medical personnel had informed them that there was no cure for Ebola. For example, some drank concentrated salt solution with the hope that it would prevent them from contracting Ebola. One of them told me that she almost died after drinking the salt solution because of her underlying high blood pressure. Some friends told me how they had been looking everywhere for bitter kola nuts and could not find any. Previously this nut was so common that one would see it everywhere one might "turn one's eyes." One told me that they had to travel to Sagamu from Lagos (about 43 miles), before they could get bitter kola nuts—and they were sold for more than five times the regular price.

When I was at the Murtala Mohammed Airport, Lagos, Nigeria, in January 2015, preparing to depart from Nigeria for the United States, I filled out an Ebola screening form and had my temperature checked with the temperature scanner before boarding the plane. On my first day at work after arriving back from Nigeria, I met two of my colleagues coming out of the door as I entered. In their attempt to avoid making contact with me they walked briskly away from the widely opened door. Upon arriving at the office, I just dropped my bag and went directly to see my mentor. She told me that I should be on self-monitoring and avoid coming in close contact with any of my colleagues for 21 days. "I expect you to act professionally," she said. Accordingly, I always sat far away from everyone at our cancer center laboratory meetings. On February 2, 2015, at one of our laboratory meetings, I still sat far away from everyone, but she told me that I had completed the 21-day self-monitoring and should be sitting close to everyone now. Nigeria had been declared Ebola-free by the WHO on October 20, 2014.

Visiting Nigeria

In the following account, Wendy Ikuomola writes in her own British style the fear expressed by her friends in the UK when she told them that she would be traveling to Nigeria. She also remembers how she had filled out the Ebola screening form at the Murtala Mohammed International Airport in Lagos, Nigeria, and gives other interesting accounts of her experience.

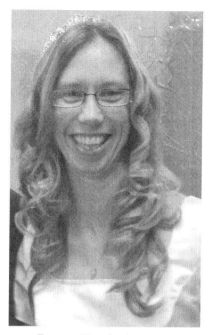

Fig. 19: Wendy Ikuomola

When I told people I was going to Nigeria the first reaction from a few people was to ask if it was safe. The connotation of Africa used to be of starving children, and in the UK especially, Band Aids song 'Feed the world.' This band released a single to raise money for the famine in Ethiopia, 1983-1985. Now, the first thought seems to be EBOLA! Would I be OK? Would I catch it and die? These were the questions I was frequently asked, especially by those close to me. I had to explain that, yes, Ebola had been in Nigeria, but the nation had acted quickly and appropriately and had eradicated it. The country had already been declared free of Ebola for some time. I felt it was one of the safest countries to go to as they had had Ebola in the country but managed it well, I tried to explain.

When at the airport leaving the UK to go out to Nigeria we had to fill in a form about our health--all to do with Ebola. It asked questions about whether we had had a high temperature recently, or been sick, or if we had been with people who had been sick? Then when we arrived at the gate to get on the aeroplane they took our temperature with a scanning thermometer. At first I didn't realize what they were doing as it hadn't been explained, but just done as I walked up to the gate. Again when we arrived in Nigeria at the passport control they took our temperature with the scanning thermometer. So they were all very vigilant and the right precautions were being taken.

Once in Nigeria, Ebola was not even thought of or mentioned again. It was only back at the airport once again to fly home that Ebola was considered again. The first thing I had to do was to fill in a form once again asking the same questions about being sick or having a high temperature. This was to be filled in either just before or just after checking in. Again my temperature was taken with a scanning thermometer. Then that seemed to be just the beginning. There were about four more checkpoints before reaching the gate, some were just the usual security checks, but there seemed to be more than usual, seeming especially to have an emphasis on health, and filling in forms and checking the temperature.

As we walked out of the aeroplane after landing back in the UK, our temperatures were taken once more.

Funnily enough, once having arrived home back in the UK no one mentioned the word Ebola to me. It was as if they had not been worried before I left the country. I am unsure as to whether this was because I had reassured them well before I left, or if they had forgotten, or assumed I was well because I was back safely.

So all in all it was a positive experience for me to see how countries can deal with a crisis of an epidemic.

Ebola Strike and Medical Doctors' Strike in Nigeria

Dr Olumide Oluwarotimi, a practicing medical doctor in Nigeria, writes about the situation in Nigeria when Ebola suddenly surfaced in Nigeria. The high index of suspicion of a patient with fever, vomiting, or cough was Ebola. He recounts how Ebola radically changed the medical practice in Nigeria.

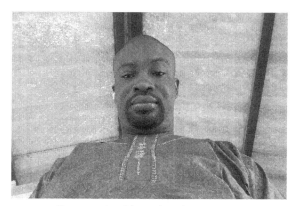

Fig. 20: Dr Olumide Oluwarotimi

Ebola disease is a deadly, hemorrhagic, disease condition caused by Ebola virus. The first case of Ebola disease was reported in Nigeria--Lagos, to be precise, on the 23rd of July 2014. When the laboratory confirmation of the country's first Ebola case was announced, the news rocked public health communities all around the world, Nigeria is Africa's most populous country and for a disease outbreak it's also a powder keg. The population of people living in Lagos is around 21million.

A Liberian-American man, Patrick Sawyer, brought the deadly Ebola virus. He was said to have been previously isolated in Liberia but escaped and traveled to Nigeria. He could travel to Nigeria easily because he was a citizen of ECOWAS. He was terribly sick when he got to Lagos Airport in Nigeria and was taken instantly to the First Consultant Hospital, Lagos for treatment. He had laboratory tests confirming that he had Ebola virus. He was abusive and wanted to escape from the hospital but the female doctor prevented him from causing more harm to the nation. The first two victims were the doctor and the nurse that managed him, it was so pathetic for the nurse had just gotten married and was pregnant. They were isolated but no one would attend to them in isolation. She had a miscarriage and no doctor wanted to do manual vacuum aspiration for her. She died of sepsis related to retained products of conception.

The most unfortunate thing during this time of national emergency was that the Nigerian Medical Association (NMA) had embarked on an indefinite strike which started on the 1st of July 2014. Because the government failed to have a genuine dialogue with the association and did not yield to the demands of the association, every attempt to end the strike proved abortive. During this period many of those that had had contacts with the victims were isolated until determination by laboratory investigation whether or not they were carrying the virus. One of the victims escaped to Port Harcourt where he was secretly managed by a doctor in a hotel. The man got well and travelled abroad but the doctor died thereafter of the illness.

On the 24th of august 2014, the Nigerian medical association ended their 56 day strike. There was panic everywhere as no preventive measures had yet been put in place to protect the health workers. Therefore, we doctors tagged every case of fever of sudden onset as a suspected case. An infrared thermometer was introduced to every institution, government parastatals, and hospital to check the temperature of patients at the time of entrance. The use of sanitizers was also introduced at this time.

About that time an incident happened in our hospital which led every patient take to their heels. A patient was brought with history of fever, mouth sores, and generalized maculo-papular rashes. We all thought that it was a typical case of Ebola. As we doctors were discussing the case, some of the health attendants overheard the discussion and, assuming that we were correct, spread the news throughout the hospital and the town. As a result, patients stopped coming to the hospital for days. After we had opportunity to obtain a proper history, we discovered that it was merely chicken pox complicated by a drug reaction.

On the 20th of October 2014, the WHO declared Nigeria an Ebola free nation. It was a spectacular success story showing that Ebola can be contained. This success story can now help many other developing countries that are deeply worried by the prospects of an imported Ebola case and are eager to improve their preparedness plans. Many wealthy countries with outstanding health systems may have something to learn as well.

Health-care delivery system in Africa

Dr. Thompson served previously as medical missionary in many parts of Africa. He remembered his experiences working in those hospitals in

Africa with limited resources. He writes in response to my request to help us understand the situation of meagre health infrastructures and medical resources in West Africa prior to Ebola outbreaks.

These are my observations, experiences and opinions regarding medical care in Africa. These experiences occurred 12-15 years ago and things have almost certainly changed since, therefore, my comments may not be as pertinent now as they might have been then.

The following experiences while in Ghana made an impression on me.

Ghana

While consulting with patients and giving health lectures in Kumasi a homeopathic doctor that was translating for me invited me to accompany him to his clinic in another town. While there I consulted on a few patients and then heard him describe his practice. He showed me an instrument with a piece of metal hanging by a string. By observing the movement of the metal he was able to determine what homeopathic medication to give to the patient. During our later conversation he volunteered to me that he didn't know if this really had any scientific basis, but since people seemed to be helped by it, he believed it was proper for him to continue the practice. I cite this example not to condemn him, but to demonstrate the quality of much of the traditional medical practice in the area.

I visited another medical clinic, and while there spent time in the pharmacy. Most of the medications were mixed, packaged, etc. in very primitive conditions without the ability to keep instruments and containers clean, to say nothing about sterile—or standardized. The clinic was very busy, and well-staffed. But quality of care was very lacking. I sympathized with the challenge the care-givers faced.

A colonel who had served with the African peace keepers in Rwanda during the genocide, invited me to go with him to his home village many miles away from Kumasi. There I met an old lady, poor, lonely, and in great need. I noticed that he took a role of bills from his pocket and placed them in her hand before bidding her farewell. We then visited an Ashanti Paramount chief in his home. It was a beautiful modern home that would have been admired even here in the states. He was responsible to the Ashanti king who shared power and authority with the civilian government, but in many ways had greater power over the people than the civilian power. He told me that he lived in New York City and had a business there. He ruled his province from there and came to Africa only occasionally for a visit. The colonel then took me to a school. I was positively impressed, because, even though there were no desks or other amenities, the kids were being educated and receiving quality meals. I suspected that his influence as a colonel in the military permitted special government favors to his village.

I visited the herbal pharmacy next door to the park where we were holding our out-door meetings. I tried to get the herbalists to share some of their secrets with me. They were not interested. Ghana is probably one of the African nations with the highest standard of living and medical care. Politics and tradition are very strong here.

Rwanda

When I arrived in Rwanda the nation was just beginning to recover from the catastrophe of the genocide. The UN was working hard to restore civility to the nation. ADRA was very active and doing a great job. The hospital at Mugonero, was once the referral center for quality medical care throughout that entire area of Africa. It had been taken over by the government during the genocide and remained so until shortly before my arrival to fill in for the medical director while he was away getting continuing education in preventive medicine. The hospital was devoid of most everything medical. We had no dependable electricity. Generators were not functioning. We had running water in the OR and did have a director of sterile supplies that did an excellent job with what he had available. The suture that I had to use for surgery was carefully selected before beginning the case from among a large bucket of donated sutures of every size, kind and age. It was difficult to find two packs the same. I scrubbed with bar soap and tap water before donning cleaned and sterilized used gloves. Anesthesia was by spinal. Our staff had experienced many changes of professional personnel since the genocide, and trusted no one—not one another, and certainly not anyone from outside as were those of us from other lands that were there to administer and render professional care.

One of the patients in the hospital when I arrived was just recovering from a rather radical debridement of rotten, retained placenta--having arrived at the hospital several days after giving birth, and having walked or been carried in a hammock from home many miles away. She was totally incontinent of urine and lay in a pool of urine continuously, but was afebrile and recovering well from the extensive surgery. Each day I saw her she begged me to repair the defect. One day I finally "gave in" to her plea against my better judgment, and took her to surgery to attempt the repair. After several hours of very difficult reconstructive surgery and many prayers, I finally placed multiple drainage catheters and closed my incision. She did surprisingly well post op. I could only praise God for His goodness in guiding my hands and judgment. Then, on the day I was scheduled to leave for home, she began leaking urine again. I was devastated—as was she. But! A couple months later, the "nurse" that had scrubbed with me on her care e-mailed me and told me that he had seen her in the out-patient clinic and that she was healed and had no more incontinence. My prayers really had been answered.

(This is a frequent problem in Africa and much of the third world, and specialists in repair are few and far between).

One evening I was called to see a small child with more that 40% burn. We had no supplies for cut-downs for I V fluids, etc., but worse than that, the "nursing" staff refused my orders and recommendations, doing things their way instead. Malaria and tuberculosis was rampant in the hospital and clinic. They claimed many lives in spite of the best efforts of the staff to contain the spread and to administer proper medications. We had no way for evaluating for AIDS at the time. I understand, and believe that many positive changes have since resulted in marked improvement in care at that facility, and in the nation.

Ile-Ife, Nigeria.

Of course you know Nigeria ever so much better than I, but permit me to share some of my experience and observations. The hospital had once been a state-of-the- art facility. When I was there as short-term medical director, it was no longer so. We had no running water in the hospital. The spring from which water had been obtained was unkempt and pipes from it to the hospital were blocked and impossible to keep open and functioning. For surgery I scrubbed with an antiseptic from a bottle. Gloves, electro cautery, gowns, and most everything else were cleaned and re-sterilized. That summer, the government was renovating the electrical system and fuel for the generator was usually unavailable, so that we were never certain to have power to do surgery, whether day or night. The hospital had a residency for training physicians, one that I was told was one of the best in the nation. It was true. They had a good theoretical grasp of the profession of medicine. But, because of inadequacies of the hospital, they had to contend with many very difficult factors that prevented them from gaining broad experience. We had endoscopes, but no technicians capable of keeping them in working order. We had many other donated instruments of all kinds, but it was difficult to find matching parts to make them functional. Just one example.

One day I needed a rigid esophageal endoscope. The patient had been at the government hospital but they did not have the instruments or expertise to remove a foreign body in the throat, so was referred to us. I found multiple scopes, but finding a light source to go with even one of them took a very long search. That procedure ended up as a success, fortunately. One of the patients on the ward had extensive wounds following massive debridement's for deep infections. He was being treated with wet-to-dry soaks, but to do so they needed to use expensive gauze sponges and sterile water from 16 ounce IV bottles obtained from Europe, costing the hospital $1.00 US each. The patient, like most, had no money, and by the time I was there, his family and friends, too, were in poverty.

A lady began to hemorrhage following a repeat C-section done by the residents when they had no supervision. We ended up taking her back to surgery, but found no identifiable source of bleeding and had to close her up still bleeding, while using all of the available bank blood and all the lab could find. She continued to bleed. The Family became very upset and demanded that we get help from the government hospital. A surgeon came, evaluated the patient, and insisted that we take her back to surgery again against my better judgment. We did, but found no single source of bleeding. We returned her to the ICU for the night (a large room with one bed, one light bulb hanging from the ceiling, and an I V stand. I slept little that night awaiting a call to pronounce her dead at any time. I received no calls. Arriving in the ICU early in the morning I discovered that she was still alive and no longer bleeding. I miraculous healing of post -partum DIC was nothing short of a miracle. I must add this comment. The hospital was later sued over the care given to this lady. Thus we see that not only is delivery of quality care always possible for many reasons, but the western practice of legal action is also beginning to challenge care as well.

One afternoon a young man was brought into the emergency department who had tried to catch a ride on a moving vehicle, missed the mark and fell by the wayside. He was in deep shock when he arrived in the E.R. When I arrived, he had a single IV in his arm and had already had two pints of fluid infused. He had no money or friends or family with money. I insisted that we load him with fluids and get him out of shock. He responded to the fluids and stabilized quite well. All of the evidence was that he was bleeding intra-abdominally and needed exploration, but the hospital administration was unable to permit this for lack of funds. In place, I ordered IV fluids as needed to maintain urine output and adequate blood pressure. Unfortunately, because of cost of I V's and other supplies, my orders were ignored and the patient died.

As already alluded to, this hospital was itself "dying" because of its attempt to provide western style care without western resources. It is unlikely that this problem will be soon resolved, but, with a bit of cultural education many of the needs could be easily corrected by using things readily available to them, and knowing how to apply them. For example: Gauze sponges could easily be made from cloth available locally for little or nothing. Families spend their days at the hospital grounds waiting around for the patients to get well, when they could just as well be put to work making the gauze into dressings ready for sterilization. I V solutions used for wet to dry dressings could be used by filtering and boiling water obtained locally, obtainable for almost nothing, thus saving the cost of sterile IV solutions for general non-IV use. Many, many are the other possible solutions to the financial problems—if only people knew how and what to do.

Chapter Eleven
New West Africa: Preventing Ebola Historical Repetition

Cultural evolution, revolution, and resolution

According to American Evaluation Association (AEA), culture is defined as "the shared experiences of people, including their languages, values, customs, beliefs, mores, worldviews, ways of knowing, and ways of communicating.[433] A viable culture is not stagnant, static, or stale but fluid, dynamic, and reciprocal.[433] Culture is dynamic when it passes through the process of "ultrafiltration" in order to be more refined. The "ultrafiltration" makes it possible to eliminate the "waste and toxic components" of the culture while preserving the best parts for optimal societal utilization. Cultural evolution takes place subtly around us as new generations easily embrace it, even while the old generations that try to restrict it.[434] Every generation defines itself through cultural evolution.[435] Cultural revolution brings drastic changes to culture through conscientious coercive efforts in order to adopt and adapt to the prevailing life situations.[436] The 18th Century industrial revolution in Europe changed the culture as an agrarian, handicapped, and handicraft economy to that of machine, technology, industry, electricity, petroleum, socioeconomics, and inventions.[437] The 1966 China cultural revolution laid more emphasis on ideological purity than on an expert management system.[438] Advancement in technology (see figure 21) is one of the social catalysts that can bring an inevitable change to a culture.[439]

The Ebola Virus and West Africa

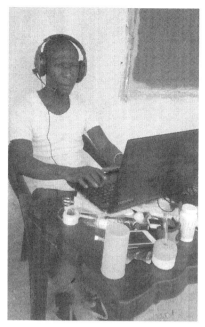

Fig. 21: Internet use in Africa

Many centuries ago in West Africa, when they wanted to communicate

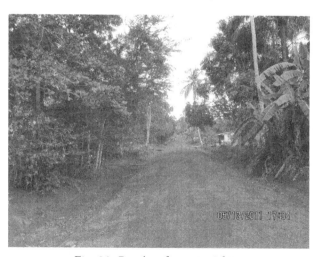

Fig. 22: Road to forest in Africa

with someone during normal daily life, or with those lost in the forest after work (see figures 22 and 23),

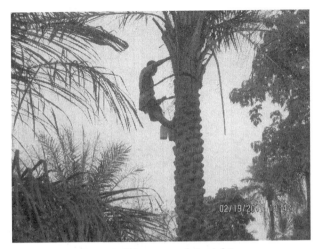

Fig. 23: Man at work in Africa

their methods of communication used were through coded beating of the talking drum (see figure 24),

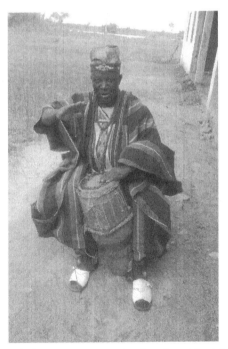

Fig. 24: Ancient communicating drum in Africa

idiophones (self-sound producing instruments), membranophones (vibration-generating membranes), music, aerophones (air column vibrating sound) incantations, and black magic.[440]

In the present generations of Africans, cellphones, the internet, and others are the fastest and best ways to communicate with anyone, even outside the sub-region[441] (see figure 25).

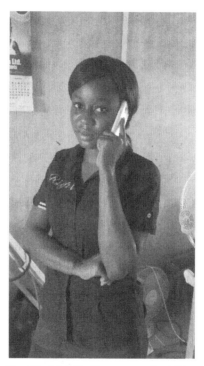

Fig. 25: Mobile Phone user in Africa

It is a cultural revolution through advanced communications and technology. In the West Africa of former days, when one walked around in the morning, one saw people using their chewing stick for cleaning the teeth (see figure 26)

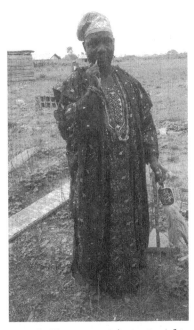

Fig. 26: Chewing stick use in Africa

but today, the majority of people (especially the younger generations) are using toothbrushes and toothpaste for dental care[442,443] (see figure 27).

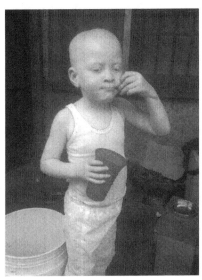

Fig. 27: Toothbrush and toothpaste use in Africa

In former times we were accustomed to using oral history as our means of passing information from one generation to the next,[444] but now people not only document through papers but by the Internet, cellphone, and other media.[445] As a matter of fact, many countries in West Africa are embracing the concept of "going green," or "going paperless." Cultural rupture often leads to cultural entropy when we fail to embrace the inevitable cultural change around us.[446] We often witness this among youth and at times label them as antisocial or as having a social misconduct behavior. In most cases it is cultural conflict that they are going through.

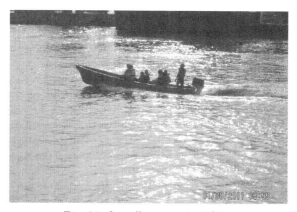

Fig. 28: Speedboat use in Africa

Before the advent of in-board and out-board engine (see figure 28), the means of transportation in the riverine areas of West Africa by way of timber log (dug-out) canoes[447] (see figure 29).

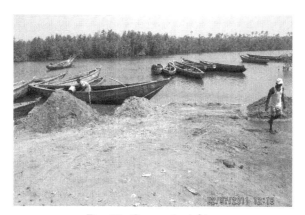

Fig. 29: Canoes in Africa

Many farmers are now using modern machines, fertilizers, and technology for farming instead of manual labor, old hoes, and machetes.[448] In the fishing industry, many West Africans are now using trawlers and other modern fishing methods[449] in place of the local fishing nets (see figure 30) and knives to catch fish.

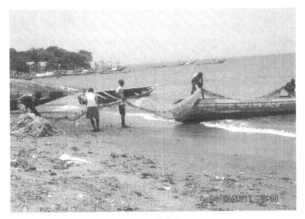

Fig. 30: Local fishing net

All these changes that we have been witnessing in West Africa happened because of a cultural resolution within us to embrace what is good and detest what is bad. There is no doubt some of these changes came through cultural evolution and, at times, cultural revolution. The most important thing to note is that we are better off now than before because we have embraced these good things. If we could change from chewing sticks to toothbrushes and toothpastes, talking drum beating to cellphone, local fishing net to modern fishing methods, and old farming methods to modern farming techniques, there is no doubt in my mind that we can still revise some of our cultural practices that enhanced the spread of Ebola and leave them behind.

In the post-Ebola West Africa (the new West Africa), we must not forget lessons that Ebola has taught us.[450] We need to unlearn some of these bad practices in our culture that allowed the Ebola outbreaks to hurt us so terribly, and to learn and re-learn[451] the aspects of ours and other's good cultures that helped us through the Ebola crises. If we fail to do this we are bound to repeat the history--and that could be even so much more devastating than what we had just experienced.

There is nothing evil in giving a befitting burial to our fallen heroes, heroines, loved ones, and families but, we can still do this without contaminating ourselves and endangering our lives. If we had to wash the corpse, we need to protect ourselves and hands with overall PPE (covering gown and gloves and others) and use disinfectant (0.5% Chlorine). We can mourn the dead without necessarily coming in contact with the body fluids of the deceased. We need to embrace safe and dignified burial practices in order to avoid transmission of diseases.[452]

It is safer to ask the person, elder statesman or elder stateswoman, heroes, heroines, or accomplished individuals to write their stories or put their knowledge or wisdom on paper, internet, or library, for the incoming generations to gain from instead of preserving their body parts. This act of documentation will provide great benefits for the next generations--not only for the continuity of knowledge,[453] but to prevent acquiring communicable diseases[454] as well. This is a cultural inheritance, not through body parts preservation, but through impacting knowledge via a durable method of knowledge transfer.[455]

Dialogue is very essential for cultural conflict resolution[456] (see figure 31). We need to employ a communal approach by engaging the community leaders, religious leaders, faith healers, or tribal chiefs in discussion--to reason with us on why we need to avoid some of the cultural practices and still show empathy for the deceased and families.[457] Safe cultural practices, especially burial, will involve training as well.[457] We need to see these people as partners in progress and not as antagonists. It is better to be engaged in a constructive dialogue process[458] which may require more than one meeting. We should also seek to know and understand the community, and to continue to create a working relationship and have informal meetings with them as well. We must help the community to understand that whatever we are doing is to increase their chances of survival, minimize spreading of disease, and to enhance their safety.[2] As the saying goes, "Nature abhors vacuum," so it is applicable in culture, "Culture abhors vacuum." If one is asking them not to do something one must also provide a satisfactory alternative before the people are found to fill a void with something even more terrible. In propounding the concept of cultural shift, we must be conversant with cultural resistance and must quickly identify and respond to it before it becomes a focus of cultural dissident dissemination.[459] We need a lot of patience to bring about cultural change.

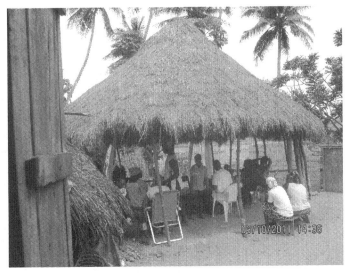

Fig. 31: Community engagement

The Ebola outbreaks in West Africa have also taught us that our cultural practices contributed directly and indirectly to Ebola spread.[1,2] The direct impacts emanated from our burial cultural practices, mourning practices, sharing (bush meat, belongings of Ebola deceased people) cultures, and togetherness (sleeping on the same bed with sick people) practices.[1,2] While indirect impacts came from our culture of corruption, bribery, centralization, negligence of health facilities and infrastructures, complacency, unpreparedness, poor governance, and lack of accountability and transparency.[20,28,460] As long as these cultural practices (direct and indirect) are not addressed it will be impossible for us to put into practice the lessons that Ebola outbreaks have taught us.[461]

We should only share food with others when we know it is safe (safe food-sharing practices). In a situation where outbreaks have been discovered, it is better to forego the culture of sharing[462] until everything is back to normal. We should also endeavor to cook the food thoroughly and in a clean environment in order to minimize contamination of the food and subsequent transmission of inherent disease in the food.[463] Our lessons from Ebola should teach us to avoid eating bat meat or coming in contact with bats[464] In the new West Africa we need to do all things possible to reduce the culture of poverty while also elevating human dignity.[465]

We can still care for our loved ones without necessarily sleeping in the same bed with them, especially when it is not safe to do so. What good will it do us if in the process of caring for someone we love we end up becoming another person to be cared and catered to? We need to understand the importance of quarantine and isolation. These are not punishments, but necessary steps that will deter wide spread infectiousness and quicken the recovery for the sick person.[466] If safe, the ashes of the cremated family members should be returned to the family members or community leaders and should be encouraged to have safe burial practices.[467] Family members must be part of the decision to cremate (or other forms of burial) Ebola corpses, and the reason for the practice must be provided and explained in detail to them. We need to also inform the families that cremation does not prevent them from still mourning for the dead.

When we fix the lessons from the Ebola outbreaks firmly in our minds, we will be able to apply them to prevent any communicable disease outbreak, to act promptly, and to control it quickly.[468] We should also communicate the desired cultural practices[469] in our schools, market places, and community town halls through posters, flyers, billboards, media, and dramatic presentations. See table 12.

Table 12: Socio-Cultural Evolution, Revolution, and Resolution

Pre-Ebola Socio-Cultural Practices	Proposed Post-Ebola Socio-Cultural Practices
Wailing or mourning and in contact with the deceased ones	Wailing or mourning without coming in contact with the deceased ones
Washing the corpse with bare hands	Washing the corpse with long-covering and double gloved PPE
Caring and kissing of the sick ones	Caring without kissing the sick ones
Sleeping on the same bed with the sick person	Avoid sleeping on the same bed with sick person

Sharing of deceased belongings	Know the cause of death of the deceased and avoid sharing if cause is infectious disease
Poorly cooked bush meat sharing	Avoid bush meat sharing especially during outbreaks. Properly cooked one can be shared when there is no outbreaks
Food stuff sharing	Infected or contaminated food stuff should not be shared
Poor hand-washing habit	Encourage good hand-washing practice
Lack of integration of traditional medicine into medical school training curriculum	Integration of traditional medicine into medical school training curriculum
Lack of efficient incorporation of traditional medicinal program	Incorporation of traditional medicinal program into National Health scheme
Keeping of parts of the bodies of heroes or heroines as a means of generational knowledge preservation and transfer	Documentation of memorable history and events as the best means of generational knowledge preservation and transfer
Poor health record system	Effective and efficient health record system
Poor communication and networks	Improved communication and networks
Centralized health care delivery system	Decentralized health care delivery system
Poor infrastructures	Improved infrastructures
Inefficient infectious surveillance program	Effective infectious surveillance program
Lack of functioning Border Health facilities	Efficient Border Health facilities
Lack of basic amenities	Provision of functioning and sustainable basic amenities
Lack of social security	Effective social security

Deficient outbreak responder training	Outbreak responder training
Lack of continual infectious training courses, workshops, and simulation exercises	Effective and continual infectious training courses, workshops, and simulation exercises
Untrained Traditional healers or faith healers as first line of health care providers	Trained traditional healers or faith healers maybe the first line of health care providers and to refer as required
Lack of cooperation between traditional healers and medical personnel	Collaborative work between trained traditional healers and medical personnel
Deficient multi-disciplinary collaboration	Efficient multi-disciplinary collaboration
Mistrust between the governors and governed	Enhanced trust between governors and governed
Ingrained culture of bribery and corruption	Minimize if not eradicate culture of bribery and corruption
Embraced culture of impunity	Need to embrace accountability and transparency policy
Inefficient professional responsibility practice	Effective professional responsibility practice
Practice of unscientific health remedies	Practice only scientific and evidence-based health remedies
Poor disease reporting system	Enhanced disease reporting system
Erratic health education program	Sustained health education program
Slow at seeking for health care	Promote prompt health-seeking behavior
Poor contact tracing technique	Improved contact tracing technique
Dwarfed health care investment	Adequate health care delivery investment
Perennial culture of poverty	Elevate beyond poverty line

Traditional healer incorporation Program

We need to face the reality, there is no way that West Africa can meet the required physician-patient ratio overnight. So, the question is, what do we do? First, we must continue to make a conscientious effort to ensure that the health personnel training continues uninterrupted.[470] Second, we need a traditional-healer program whereby we can study what traditional healers know and what they are doing so as to be able to advise them on safe traditional African medicinal practices[471] (Note: traditional African medicinal practitioners include the faith healers, herbalists, traditional healers, and birth attendants). We need to help them understand their limitations and when to call for help or to refer cases. We need to work hand-in-hand with them. We cannot just turn a blind eye to the reality of our times, for the majority of West Africans are seeking help from the Traditional medicinal practitioners--even before consulting the professional health personnel.[472] It cannot be denied that there continues to be a high level of trust in traditional African medicinal practice in some parts of our community.[471, 472] We need to give them training in effective hand-washing, disinfectant use, making simple diagnosis, applying safe hygienic practices, environmental cleanliness, and safe and good traditional medicinal practices in general.[471, 472] We may classify them as Alternative Medicine Practitioners as it is being done in China, UK, and other parts of the world.[474] They must obtain continuing education (training) in order to update their knowledge and upgrade their tools.[471,472] They need to be affiliated with a nearby health facility where referrals from them can be attended to and where for monitoring of them can be done to ensure that they are complying with safe traditional African medicinal practices. We can learn social medicine[473] and herbs from them. We can also conduct research on some of the herbs they are using.

Integration of African traditional health into Medical curriculum

In order to efficiently and effectively work with the traditional African medicinal practitioners, the medical school curriculum must also include information as to what traditional African medicinal practice is and how it works, its strengths, and limitations.[475] It is also advisable that community health posting (rotations) include opportunities to work with the traditional African medicinal practitioners.[476] This type of symbiotic or mutual relationship and professionalism will erase the biases that exist between the two as well foster a formidable working relationship for the good of the society[477] of West Africa.

Professional responsibility in fighting Ebola outbreaks

5 Ps (Personal, peers, public, policy, and patriotism): In moving forward from the Ebola epidemic to the New West Africa, there are some professional responsibilities we need to reflect on and take with us always. See Fig. 32.

Personal

Our personal protection is not only important for us and our family but to prevent us from us spreading diseases to others as well.[478] PPE is very important for preventing transmission of communicable diseases to others.[478] It is also very germane that we take personal responsibility for whatever we are doing. We need to be trustworthy and be trusted. When one makes a mistake we need to accept it as one's fault and inform the necessary authority about it. We must avoid falsification, fraud, and irresponsible behaviors.[479] I remember working with some health personnel who often used the hospital's ketamine injection for themselves. I also remember how another health worker used the diazepam tablets of the health facility. We need to seek for help when we find ourselves in these conditions.

Peers

One needs to be conscious of the fact that we are also obligated to our peers to see that they are as well protected by the decisions and the behavior we engage in as we are.[480] When things go wrong in the medical field, everyone is being looked upon as "birds of the same feathers fly together." In whatever we are doing, we need to consider our impact upon our peers and colleagues as well. If we know we have contracted a communicable disease, we need to quarantine or isolate ourselves so that our peers and family are not unnecessarily exposed to what we have contracted.[481] As it is being said, "if you see something say something," this is only way to contact trace, and prevent further spreading of communicable diseases.

Public

Our professional responsibility exacts that we provide health education as well as to protect the public from contagious diseases.[482] In order to prevent communicable diseases from spreading to the public at large, we need to quarantine and isolate, report outbreaks immediately, and instigate instant contact tracing.[481, 482] Bad news from irresponsibly professional behavior goes viral in the public and it usually takes a long time to fade away.

Policy

Policy makers must have a contingency fund by which they can adequately, promptly, and sufficiently rise to the occasion.[483] We saw what happened in the three badly affected countries in West Africa. They did not have anything for such an eventuality.[484] The health ministry or department must have high a level of preparedness in order to avoid being found wanting whenever there is any clarion call to actions. It is not necessary to wait until an outbreak occurs before instituting a surveillance program.[485] An on-going surveillance program will make it possible for a communicable disease to be detected early and provisions made whereby to provide the necessary remedy. It should be standard operational procedure (SOP) to have disinfectants in the health facility and to assure that health personnel always comply with good hygiene procedures. We should continue to incorporate updated policy of WHO, CDC, or organizations such as MSF into our preventative measures against communicable diseases.

Patriotism

Our primary constituency is the medical community. Following Physician's Hippocratic Oath demands some level of patriotism and faithfulness.[486] Citizenship to any nation also requires us to be patriotic.[487] This means, as health personnel, that double patriotism is required of us. Being patriotic leads us to be more dedicated, determined, devoted, and diligent. These are attributes that are needed on the medical battle field in order to fight and win the communicable diseases war. Patriotism makes me want to protect myself with PPE,[1,2] prevent my peers from being infected, protect the public, promote public health, and join advocacy groups to ensure that policy is formulated and complied with.

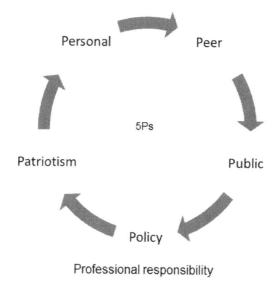

Fig. 32

West African Health Organization (WAHO)

In 1987 WAHO was formed by the heads of the governments of the 15 countries of ECOWAS with the following visions and strategies:[488]

- Maintaining sustainable partnerships
- Strengthening capacity building
- Collecting, interpreting and disseminating information
- Promoting cooperation and ensuring coordination and advocacy
- Exploiting information communication technologies.

WAHO has nine programs which are expected to fulfill the organization's missions and strategies: [488,489]

- Coordination and harmonization of policies
- Health information
- Development of research
- Promotion and dissemination of best practices
- Development of human resources for health
- Medicines and vaccines
- Traditional medicine

- Diversification of health financing mechanisms
- WAHO institutional development and capacity building program

As with most of the programs and organizations in West Africa, lack of funds, lack of transparency and accountability, bribery, and corruption have eroded public trust and confidence of the donors to continue financing them.[490-492] It was so obvious that WAHO could not do much when Ebola struck at its borders.[493] It was created to prevent outbreaks such as Ebola and also to protect the citizens of the sub-region from other communicable diseases. Unfortunately, WAHO was overpowered by Ebola.

If WAHO is going to be relevant to the people of West Africa and able to meet the enormous challenges in the sub-region, it needs to be privatized. It will do better under privatization[494] than under the ECOWAS which are saddled not only with bureaucracy, but lack of transparency, commitment, and underfunding as well.[490-492]

A new WAHO should be proactive and have rapid responders that will respond immediately to any future outbreaks in the region.[495] It should also have a database that will monitor and track all health-related events in the sub-region. Health data and information sharing about any communicable diseases and outbreaks should be hitch-free among the countries in the sub-region.[488] WAHO should encourage various countries in the sub-region to spend more on health than now and to fund surveillance and public health programs. There should be high level of preparedness always. WAHO should also encourage the West African government to fund research and health care delivery systems.

Outbreak responder training

The government in the sub-region should have a curriculum in their health schools for dealing with outbreaks. Specifically, this this curriculum must include both the common and the rare infectious diseases. The training should include the dissemination of information for community health as well. Having a program like this will not only enhance patient safety but also reduce unemployment rates among the youth.[28] It is not right to continue to try to solve 21st Century problems with 19th Century solutions. The rate at which the populations in West Africa is exploding is faster than the rate of job creation and employment.[496] According to UNICEF population projections, by mid-Century, Africa will be home to 41% of the world births, and by the end of this Century four out of every ten of the world populations will be Africans.[496] This is another Ebola lessons. Let us provide outbreak responding courses in our health institutions and train our youth on how to respond along with basic hygiene practice, community health education, basic health knowledge, and cultural-health education.

Basic amenities and infrastructure improvement

The Ebola outbreaks in West Africa have taught us that we cannot neglect basic amenities and infrastructures in the communities, slums, and rural areas and expect excellent results. This is just a pure lesson of physics "Action and reaction are equal and opposite." We need to invest in our basic amenities and infrastructures if we do not want history of epidemics to be our eternal plight.[497] We have never learned our lessons from social conflicts and wars that wrecked the sub-region because of the lack of development in some areas. At times when citizens of those undeveloped areas have felt neglected they have taken on arms to fight for their rights.[28] We cannot expect improvement for future generations so long as the majority of our populations live in abject poverty. The mathematics does not add up that way. How can we expect people to wash their hands when they do not even have water in their homes? Some of these people have to walk many miles to the stream in order to get water for the family to use for bathing, drinking, and cooking.[498] It is not too expensive to make a bore hole where water will be easily accessibility to the people.[498] Then when we demonstrate to them hand-washing for preventing Ebola and other contact-spreading communicable diseases; it will be easier to do. If we really want the governed to trust the governors or governments,[499] it will have to begin by investing in the basic amenities and infrastructures required by the people. By this, they know someone cares. In return, they will also care enough to trust the government and listen to its health messages. It is true that the governments have not listened to the people[499] that told the politicians what they needed before they voted for them. Therefore, it should be no surprise that during the Ebola crises the people paid the governments back in their own coins in failing to trust the health message they were telling them. More so, the governed in West

Africa can see the expensive cars, luxurious lives, and flamboyant parties the government officers often engage in while the people that voted for them are languishing in hunger and poverty.[500,501] In West Africa the only lucrative job is joining the winning political party and working in a government setting.[502] This mentality of embezzlement and impunity[502] must stop if we are to move past Ebola outbreaks and apply the lessons we have learned at such a high price and see the dawn of a new era in West Africa.

Decentralization

Health care delivery systems in West Africa need to be decentralized[503] if we expect to have a break-through from cyclic diseases, high mortality, and outbreaks. We do not have good roads, air ambulances, or communication systems that could have worked well in a centralized system. In the kind of terrain existing in West Africa, decentralization of our health care delivery system[504] could be a round peg in a round hole. It could save many lives and encourage prompt health management.

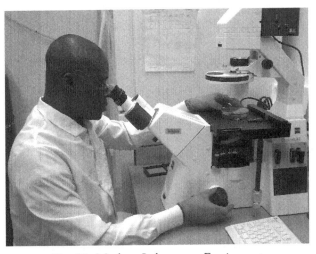

Fig. 33: Modern Laboratory Equipment

Rapid Ebola test kits

There are very few high quality laboratories or high tech laboratory personnel (see figures 33 and 34) in West Africa, so in order to keep surveillance alive in our fight against Ebola, and prevent another disastrous outbreak, the availability and accessibility of Rapid Ebola test kits[505] with high sensitivity and high specificity will be of great importance. With rapid Ebola test kits, there is no need for sophisticated laboratory equipment in order to do the initial testing. It does not also require lengthy training in in order to perform the test.

Training courses, workshops, and simulation exercises

In order to make good the lessons we learned from the Ebola outbreaks, we need to redirect and re-orientate our medical curriculum and program by putting more emphasis on communicable and preventable diseases.[488] We need further training in infectious diseases that should be followed periodically with in-courses in prevention and control of communicable diseases. There should be regular workshops and information sharing among the health facilities in each country.[506] The refreshment training should also include the means for prompt recognition of potential outbreaks and the appropriate actions to be taken. There should be regular simulation exercises that should be dramatized in order to further help understand how to recognize, what to do, and who to contact.[506]

Border Health facilities

West African borders should have health facilities with health personnel that have sound knowledge in communicable diseases.[488] The border screening for Ebola should continue and should also include screening for other communicable diseases such as tuberculosis, measles, polio and others.[488] We must do all we can to minimize, if not eradicate, all these communicable diseases from West Africa. This vicious cycle of poverty and diseases must not continue within us forever. That is one of the lessons Ebola had taught us: Be prepared and be proactive![507] When we have border health facilities with knowledgeable health officers that are working along with the border control or immigration officers it will become easier for us to identify those with communicable diseases and to quarantine them.[508] From Ebola we learned that outbreaks around the rural settlements are more difficult to control, contact-trace, and quarantine than those that happened in the cities with more efficient mobile technologies and health facilities.[288,509] These border health facilities would be providing health care for those living around the borders. The border health officers would be involved in community health education which would center on basic hygiene and prompt reporting of diseases to the health facilities.[488] The border health personnel will also work with the community leaders, faith healers, traditional healers, and local chiefs. Disease surveillance, prevention, and control is a collaborative and cooperative measure which no one can do alone. A successful public health outcome starts with the ability to educate and prepare the people before a disease outbreak rather than when an outbreak is already present and people are already panicking and no longer able to comprehend instructions given to them.

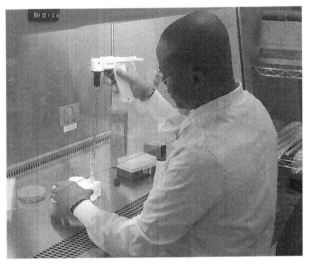

Fig. 34: Well Equipped Laboratory

Basic Approach to getting things done successfully in Africa

Africa is a very fertile continent with a many opportunities and possibilities. In spite of various factors that have plagued and continue to plague the continent, Africa remains the beacon of beauty, cradle of civilization, and the source of developmental materials and mineral resources. Africans are very receptive people with sunshine-like love and warm hearts, a sterling characteristic that is impossible for poverty to impoverish. In dealing with Africans and in Africa, the basic approach to get things done successfully is very important, a neglect of this basic and simple approach could result in poor outcome and frustration. The acronym is called **C-CULTURE-ES.**

Culture: The gateway to the African Continent is to seek to understand the culture of the people. Africa is a unique continent with a strong sense of culture and tradition. By endeavoring to understand the culture, it will help one to see Africans through the lens of their culture, thereby putting one in a better position to have a meaningful interaction with them. As previously noted, culture is the centerpiece of the life in Africa--even the Africans in diaspora. In Africa, there is culture of hierarchy, younger generations are expected to revere older folks, and the older generations are expected to mentor and protect the younger ones. There is culture of care where every child is your child and one should be there for them even when the parents are not there. The younger generations are expected to care for their parents and elderly ones since most of African society has no nursing homes for the elderly. It is still considered as a taboo in most African society to fail to cater and care for your parents or elderly ones in the community, so putting them in a nursing homes is viewed as a form of neglect. Part of the culture in Africa is top-down fashion where a father is seen as the head of the family and any decision passes through him. In the same vein, in Africa, every society has a head, a representative, or leader, and it is expected that if anything is going to be done for the community, the leader must first be approached. No matter how good the intention or the project might be, bypassing this cultural hierarchical structure may lead to resistance and refusal.

Communication: This very important in African culture. Through communication, there may be community engagement, dialogue, planning, and resolution. Traditionally, Africa is a continent of oral history, so communication is vital. Communication breeds clarity and clarity yields to unambiguity. Even with the best project, if it is not properly and clearly articulated and communicated, it may result in suspiciousness.

Understanding: Being able to understand how people look at things in Africa may resolve many bottleneck problems that arise between the society and its governing organizations. It is important for the governing body to understand what the people really need--not just what it wants to do for them. What the organization thinks the people want may not be what they really need. If the organization would take the time to understand the plights of the people and why some things are being done by them the way they are being done, it would often constitute a watershed moment in passing the message across and creating a people-driven project outcome.

Look-Listen-Learn: Even as an African, this look-listen-learn phenomenon has contributed in no small measure to the way I have conducted my medical practice in some of the African countries. We engage our eye and ear senses to observe things and people around us, and then apply our minds to these observations. Africans love visitors and through your intensive and conscientious interactions with them one will understand the dos and the don'ts of the society, thus paving way for a brilliant achievement by the people conducting the project.

Togetherness: Togetherness is a classical identity of Africa. It permeates everything we do. We are a Continent of togetherness. It is an inclusive society. This togetherness and inclusiveness may be seen in the family, the community, and the religion. Unfortunately, selfish politicking is tearing our togetherness heritage apart. Fortunately, when one enters the rural dwelling, he will see that this togetherness heritage remains almost intact. So when health matters, business, or other projects are to be done, it is wise to ensure that the venture projects and promotes the spirit of togetherness that is the core of African society. Whatever the project, the more we do involve the people and avoid exclusion of the people, the greater will be their participation.

Umpteenth: A one-time dialogue is not sufficient. There is always a need for multiple times to have conversations. The first meeting may serve for setting the pace for subsequent ones. In this meeting it is important to present the salient reasons for contacting the community in a nutshell. For example, if the purpose for contacting the community is in regards to health, especially behavioral modification or cultural change, it would be well to systematically explain the difference between the new, proposed practice, and the old so that people can see the difference between two. It should be tailored towards the community means of resolving problems.

Respect: African society is anchored around respect. In demonstrating that one does respect the people of Africa, various options regarding an issue should be given and clearly explained, and then permit them to make the final decision. Any attempt to force things down their throats may result in strong resistance and hostility. Of course, respect gives rise to respect, so if the community of people are respected, one will in turn get respect from them. An aspect of respect appreciated by Africans is the honor of being kept informed from the outset, and being given the opportunity to ask questions and offer their opinions on things. This will make them feel dignified and will open the door to further possible discussion. There is no doubt that Africans learned from the history of what happened to the continent in the past but they still believe that one cannot use the theory of "one-size-fits-all" to judge everyone. Surely, people are suspicious! At the same time, they know that there may be a silver lining around every cloud! Therefore, even this barrier can be broken through genuine respect for their fundamental human rights, community rights, and personal rights.

Empathy: It is not enough to sympathize with the people of Africa. Empathy is also important. Africans are not desirous of immediate relief of their needs only, but to be taught how to prevent the thing that caused the problem in the first place, and how to manage it if they should be found in the same situation again. They do not want to be dependent forever. Such is not the spirit of entrepreneurship. They want to be partners as well. They want to be givers instead of full-time takers. Therefore, when one goes to Africa to help, one should go beyond just providing "fish" for them to eat, but in providing the materials for "fishing" and teaching them how to "fish"-and how to solve "fishing-related" problems. Such is true partnership and such is true empathy. Whatever assistance puts Africa in a perpetually dependent position is not empathy, but sympathy. So long as sympathy remains the modus operandi the vicious cycle of dependence will remain unbroken—even as long as time endures.

Expectation: It is well to ask the people of Africa what they expect from whatever intervention, assistance, or enterprise is being offered to them. On the other hand, it is also prudent to tell the people of Africa the expectation of the organization. The two expectations should then be weighed, differences discussed, and common ground attained. Of course, the expectation we set should be reasonable and achievable. For example, in addressing the issue of cultural change, the community should be made aware of what went wrong with their cultural settings, the expected characteristics of the intended modification, and why it should be preferred over the old being left behind. Possible risks, benefits, and burdens they may have to bear in the course of their participation need to be included in the discussion.

Strategy: Strategy should be a community, people-oriented strategy that has full understanding and input of the people. Africans prefer the thought that, "This is our thing" to "This is their thing." If it is considered, "This is our thing," they will go all out to ensure that it is successful. The strategy should include both short-term and long-term approaches, with interim and periodic analyses, evaluations, and monitoring. The strategy should be age, education, language, and culture appropriate such as may appeal to the majority of the community. The greater the inclusion of the targeted population, the greater the degree of participation and success to be expected. In addition to the above, strategy should also be flexible to give room for any contingency or unexpected situation.

Chapter Twelve
Conclusion

It is very important that African cultural medicine be well understood if one hopes to prevent a cultural clash with modern Western medical practice. No matter how promising a proposed change may appear as a benefit for the people, unless one understands the African culture and is willing to work with that culture, one may expect only detestation and rejection of the proposal.[510]

In keeping with the Hippocratic Oath, "to do no harm," taken by physicians, understanding the African culture will not only help to prevent professional medical personnel from doing harm or experiencing modern medicine-African cultural conflict, it will, rather, help medical health care givers to embrace the positive aspects of African culture while at the same time gradually eliminating some of the most dangerous African cultural practices.[510, 511]

Ebola is a medico-cultural disease. The Ebola outbreaks in West Africa attest to the medico-cultural junction that exists between medical management, prevention, control, and prognosis, and those cultural practices that spread the disease and hinder prompt containment.

In order to say "Never Again" to Ebola in West Africa, we need to understand the role socio-cultural factors play in the Ebola's acquisition and transmission. Understanding these socio-cultural factors may facilitate the development of those management measures necessary to respond to and resist the lethal threat of Ebola, i.e. identifying suspicious cases; establishing the diagnosis; applying prompt and effective treatment; willingness to be isolated and quarantined; reporting suspicious cases; contact tracing; participating in surveillance operations; and complying with preventive directives. "Never again" can only be truly "Never again" when we make use of the lessons we have learned from this debilitating disease.

The comprehensive impact of Ebola in West Africa may take many years to fully comprehend. However, there is no doubt that the immediate impact has led to reductions in population, GDP, health infrastructures, health personnel, tourism, and foreign reserves, and to increases in the number of orphans, governmental spending, poverty, and dependence.

Because of the effects of the Ebola on the economies of West Africa, it would not only be difficult to fight another outbreak of Ebola, but of any other communicable or costly non-communicable disease as well. In championing a new course for West Africa in the post-Ebola era, we must not only incorporate cultural modification into our system; but we must adopt and adapt a cultural revolution to deal with culture-enhancing diseases and conditions in our society. Our biggest challenge during the intra-Ebola crisis in West Africa was our culture. Culture was one of the primary obstacles that made us so vulnerable to Ebola disease. In view of this fact, clinging to the same cultural practices that brought woes on us would be tantamount to self-destruction. A lesson is not learned if it does not effect a positive change in the society.

Africa is a religious continent. As enumerated in chapter three, there are many kinds of religions in African society. They all have one thing in common, they encourage their followers to hope for the best as they cope with the worst. The Christian leaders among them also implore their followers to have a blessed hope in the second return of Jesus Christ where He will establish eternal life and there will be no suffering, pain, death, or Ebola disease. We can build on this African rich culture of hopefulness as we deal with the Ebola hopelessness. We can encourage the African society to be hopeful for better days ahead as we slowly settle down to a life without Ebola in Africa.

Our resources are great, spanning the entire gamut of culture—from physical to deeply spiritual. But as we have witnessed throughout the Ebola crisis, the good and the evil are often seen to be in conflict. The love that exists in the heart of every human being too often yields to the selfishness that strives against it. As a result, our cultural resources, as great as they may be, will fail unless they are not selfishly used for the advancement of the society.

Surely, it requires time, patience, funds, and hope to cope with the devastating effects of Ebola in a post-Ebola era in Africa. It is time for us to come and bring our resources together, not only to prevent another Ebola crisis or other communicable disease, but to strategize, protect, prepare, and equip our health sector for the 21st Century and beyond.

NB: Liberia was declared Ebola free on May 9, 2015.

List of Abbreviations

5Ps	Personal, peers, public, policy, and patriotism
AIDS	Acquired immune deficiency syndrome
ASEOWA	African Union Support to Ebola Outbreak in West Africa
AU	African Union
C-CULTURE-ES	Culture, Communication, Understanding, Look-Listen-Learn, Togetherness, Umpteenth, Respect, Empathy, Expectation, Strategy
CDC	Centers for Disease Control and Prevention
DIC	Disseminated intravascular coagulation
DRC	Democratic Republic of Congo
ECOWAS	Economic Community of West Africa States
ELISA	Enzyme-linked immunosorbent assay
ER	Emergency room
ETU	Ebola treatment unit
EVD	Ebola virus disease
FAO	Food and Agriculture Organization
FDA	Food and Drug Administration
FGM	Female genital mutilation
GDP	Gross domestic product
HIV	Human immunodeficiency virus
ICU	Intensive care unit
IDRC	International Development Research Centre
IgG	Immunoglobulin G
IgM	Immunoglobulin M
ILO	International Labour Organization
IPC	Infection Prevention Control
IV	Intravenous
JFK	John F. Kennedy
MSF	Medecins Sans Frontieres (Doctors without borders)

NCI	National Cancer Institute
NGO	Non-governmental organization
NIH	National Institutes of Health
NMA	Nigerian Medical Association
PCR	Polymerase chain reaction
PPE	Personal protective equipment
RNA	Ribonucleic acid
RT-PCR	Reverse transcriptase polymerase chain reaction
VHF	Viral hemorrhagic fever
UN	United Nations
UNDP	United Nations Development Programme
UNESCO	United Nations Educational, Scientific and Cultural Organization
UNFPA	United Nations Population Fund
UNICEF	United Nations Children's Fund
WAHO	West Africa Health Organization
WHO	World Health Organization

Bibliography

1. Centers for Disease Control and Prevention. (2015). Outbreaks Chronology: Ebola Virus Disease http://www.cdc.gov/vhf/ebola/outbreaks/history/chronology.html
2. World Health Organization. (2014). Ebola virus disease. Retrieved from http://www.who.int/mediacentre/factsheets/fs103/en/
3. World Health Organization. (1978). Ebola haemorrhagic fever in Zaire, 1976. Report of an International Convention. Bulletin of the World Health Organization, 56(2), 271-293.
4. Brown, R. (2014, July 17). The virus detective who discovered Ebola in 1976. Retrieved from http://www.bbc.com/news/magazine-28262541
5. Baize, S., Pannetier, D., Oestereich, L., Rieger, T., Koivogui, L., Magassouba N.,… Günther, S. (2014). Emergence of Zaire Ebola virus disease in Guinea. N Engl J Med., Oct 9, 371(15), 1418-1425.
6. Centers for Disease Control and Prevention. (2013). Viral Hemorrhagic Fevers. Retrieved from http://www.cdc.gov/ncidod/dvrd/spb/mnpages/dispages/vhf.htm
7. World Health Organization. (2014). Haemorrhagic fevers, Viral. Retrieved from http://www.who.int/topics/haemorrhagic_fevers_viral/en/
8. iNaturalist.org. (n.d.). Flying foxes. Retrieved from http://www.inaturalist.org/taxa/40870-Pteropus
9. British Broadcasting Corporation. (2015). Nature wildlife: Fruit bats (Pteropus). Retrieved from http://www.bbc.co.uk/nature/life/Pteropus
10. Donnelley, P. (2014). Ebola outbreak sweeping West Africa started with two-year-old boy infected by a fruit bat, say researchers. Retrieved from http://www.dailymail.co.uk/news/article-2733122/Ebola-outbreak-sweeping-West-Africa-started-two-year-old-boy-infected-fruit-bat-say-researchers.html
11. Worldbank.org. (2014, October 8). The Economic Impact of the 2014 Ebola Epidemic: Short and Medium Term Estimates for West Africa. Retrieved from http://www.worldbank.org/en/region/

afr/publication/the-economic-impact-of-the-2014-ebola-epidemic-short-and-medium-term-estimates-for-west-africa
12. Phillips, C. J. (2005). Health economics: An introduction for health professionals, pp. 41-70. Malden, MA: Blackwell Publishing.
13. Worldbank.org. (2015, January 12). Ebola Hampering Household Economies across Liberia and Sierra Leone. Retrieved from http://www.worldbank.org/en/news/press-release/2015/01/12/ebola-hampering-household-economies-liberia-sierra-leone
14. King, J. W. (2014). Ebola Virus Infection Differential Diagnoses. Retrieved from http://emedicine.medscape.com/article/216288-differential
15. World Health Organization. (2015). Ebola Situation Report-1 April 2015. Retrieved from http://apps.who.int/ebola/current-situation/ebola-situation-report-1-april-2015-0
16. Medicins Sans Frontieres. (2015). Ebola. Retrieved from http://www.msf.org/diseases/ebola
17. Mayo Clinic Staff. (2014). Ebola virus and Marburg virus: Complications. Retrieved from http://www.mayoclinic.org/diseases-conditions/ebola-virus/basics/complications/con-20031241
18. Central Intelligence Agency. (n.d.). The world factbook: Africa. Retrieved from https://www.cia.gov/library/publications/the-world-factbook/wfbExt/region_afr.html
19. Economic Community of West Africa States. (2015). ECOWAS member states. Retrieved from http://www.ecowas.int/
20. Parry, J. K. & Ryan, A. S. (Eds.). (1995). A Cross-Cultural Look at Death, Dying, and Religion, 145-159, 160-171. Chicago, IL: Nelson-Hall.
21. Akintubuwa, O. (2014). African culture, the dead, and the living and spiritual connection (Unpublished).
22. Strong, L. (2001). African-American Ancestors: A Unique Christian Concept of Life After Death, Written works. Retrieved from http://www.mythicarts.com/writing/African_American_Ancestors.html
23. Okeke, T. C., Anyaehie, U. S. B., & Ezenyeaku, C. C. K. (2012). An Overview of Female Genital Mutilation in Nigeria. Ann Med Health Sci Res., Jan-Jun, 2(1): 70–73.
24. NHS.org. (n.d.). Female genital mutilation. Retrieved from http://www.nhs.uk/conditions/female-genital-mutilation/pages/introduction.aspx

25. Desai, M. (2009). Women Cross-Border Traders: Rethinking global trade. Development, 52, 377–386. doi:10.1057/dev.2009.29
26. United Nations Development Programme. (2014, December 30). UNDP to help cut cross border Ebola infections in West Africa. Retrieved from http://www.undp.org/content/undp/en/home/presscenter/articles/2014/12/30/undp-to-help-cut-cross-border-ebola-infections-in-west-africa-.html
27. Frimpong, P. (2014, December 14). Unemployment in Africa: What Policy Makers Should Know..., Feature article. Retrieved from http://www.modernghana.com/news/435566/1/unemployment-in-africa-what-policy-makers-should-k.html
28. Annan, N. (2014). Violent Conflicts and Civil Strife in West Africa: Causes, Challenges and Prospect. International Journal Stability of Security & Development, 3(1), 3, 1-16.
29. United Nations Educational, Scientific and Cultural Organization. (2009-2014). Literacy and non-formal education. Retrieved from http://www.unesco.org/new/en/dakar/education/literacy/
30. Lutz, W. & Samir, K. C. (2013). Demography and human development: Education and population projections. UNDP Human Development Report Office: Occasional Paper 2013/04.
31. Schultz, T. P. 1993. Mortality decline in the low-income world: Causes and consequences. American Economic Review 83(2), pp. 337-342.
32. Mensch, B., Lentzner, H., & Preston, S. (1985). Socioeconomic differentials in child mortality in developing countries. ST/ESA/SER.A/97. United Nations, New York.
33. Awolalu, J. O. (1976, Spring). What is African Traditional Religion? Studies in Comparative Religion, 10(2).
34. Mbiti, J. S. (1969). African Religions and Philosophy, Heineman, 1969, 1-10.
35. Olupona, J. K., & Nyang, S. S. (Eds.). (1993). Religious Plurality in Africa: Essays in Honour of John S. Mbiti, 68-80 Berlin: Mouton de Gruyter.
36. Akresh, R., Bhalotra, S., Leone, M., & Osili, U. O. (2012). War and Stature: Growing Up during the Nigerian Civil War. American Economic Review, 102(3), 273-277.
37. Liberia Truth and Reconciliation Commission. (2009). Preliminary Findings and Recommendations, Vol. 1.

38. Sierra Leone Truth and Reconciliation Commission. (2004). Witness to truth: report of the Sierra Leone Truth and Reconciliation Commission, vol. 3B
39. Africa Renewal. (2010 August). For African business, ending corruption is 'priority number one': UN Global Compact urges companies to operate ethically. Retrieved from http://www.un.org/africarenewal/magazine/august-2010/african-business-ending-corruption-%E2%80%98priority-number-one%E2%80%99
40. Atuobi, S. M. (2007). Corruption and State Instability in West Africa: An Examination of Policy Option. Kofi Annan International Peacekeeping Training Centre, Accra, Ghana.
41. Richmond, Y. & Gestrin, P.(2009). Into Africa: A Guide to Sub-Saharan Culture and Diversity (2nd ed.). Boston, MA: Intercultural Press.
42. Dia, M. (1993). A Governance Approach to Civil Service Reform in Sub-Saharan. World Bank Technical Paper 225 Africa Technical Department Series
43. Aminzade, R. (2013). Race, Nation, and Citizenship in Post-Colonial Africa: The Case of Tanzania, 260-261. NY, NY: Cambridge University Press.
44. Olukoshi, A. O. (1998). The Politics of Opposition in Contemporary Africa, 161-163. Stockholm: Elanders Gotab.
45. Prinsloo, M. & Breier, M. (1996). The Social Uses of Literacy: Theory and Practice in Contemporary South Africa, 12-15. Cape Town: John Benjamins Publishing Co.
46. Annan, K. (2013, July 19). Tackle tax evasion to fuel Africa's development. The Elders. Retrieved from http://theelders.org/article/tackle-tax-evasion-fuel-africas-development
47. Urbach, J. (2013 July, 15). Flat tax rate is key to economic growth. The Star Africa Edition. Retrieved from http://www.iol.co.za/news/flat-tax-rate-is-key-to-economic-growth-1.1547223#.VP3xZdE5DIU
48. Andrew, G. & Neyapti Bilin, N. (1999). Development Centre Studies Conflict and Growth in Africa, 3. Development Center Studies.
49. Zewde, B.Society, (2008). State, and Identity in African History. Forum for Social Studies.
50. Mabogunje, A. L. (n.d.). Land reform in Nigeria: Progress, problems & prospects.

51. Pedro, A. M. A. (n.d.). Mainstreaming Mineral Wealth in Growth and Poverty Reduction Strategies. An Economic Commission for Africa (ECA) Policy Paper.
52. Bekker, J. C. (1991). Nepotism, corruption and discrimination: a predicament for a post-apartheid South African public service. Politiken, 18(2), 55-73.
53. World Health Organization. (2014, August 25). Unprecedented number of medical staff infected with Ebola. Media centre. Situation assessment. http://www.who.int/mediacentre/news/ebola/25-august-2014/en/
54. Palmer, B. (2014, March 13). Should It Really Take 14 Years to Become a Doctor? It's time to experiment with medical school.
55. Chimanikire, D. P. (2005). Brain drain: Causes, and economic consequences for Africa. African Association for Public Administration and Management.
56. Feldman, R. (2012, November-December). Africa's brain drain its impacts on security and stability. Military review, 48-56.
57. Afri-Dev.info. (2014). Ebola epidemic and human resources for health challenges: 2014 Africa Factsheet on Health Workforce. Retrieved from http://www.afri-dev.info/scorecards
58. Boozary, A. S., Farmer, P. E., & Jha, A. K. (2014). The Ebola Outbreak, Fragile Health Systems, and Quality as a Cure. JAMA, 312(18), 1859-1860.
59. Rid, A. Ezekiel J. Emanuel, E. J. (2014). Why Should High-Income Countries Help Combat Ebola? JAMA, 312(13), 1297-1298.
60. Schnidman, A. (2006). The Global Effects of the Brain Drain on Health Care Systems. GUJHS, 3(1).
61. Collins, S. P. K. (2014, October 20). Liberia's 'Brain Drain' is thwarting its efforts to stop Ebola.
62. Kentikelenis, A., Lawrence King, L., McKee, M., & Stuckler, D. (2014, December 21). The International Monetary Fund and the Ebola outbreak. The Lancet Global Health, 3(2).
63. Africlandpost.com. (2015, February 13). Africa: Doctors brain drain.
64. Clottey, E. A. (2014, October 28). Confronting Ebola in West Africa. The African angle. World Plocy blog.
65. Cadei, E. (2014, December 9). Officials hope to use Ebola to build Africa's health care capabilities. http://www.npr.org/2014/12/09/369559355/officials-hope-to-use-ebola-to-build-africas-health-care-capabilities

66. American Anthropological Association. (2014, November 18). Strengthening West African Health Care Systems to Stop Ebola: Anthropologists Offer Insights.
67. Spaan, E., Mathijssen, J., Tromp, N., McBain, F., ten Have, A., & Baltussen, R. (2012). The impact of health insurance in Africa and Asia: a systematic review. Bulletin of the World Health Organization, 90:685-692
68. Afri-Dev.info. (2013). (Post Abuja+12) 2013 Africa health financing scorecard – Featuring year 2000 to 2010 indicative progress summary
69. Madamombe, I. (2006). Traditional healers boost primary health care: Reaching patients missed by modern medicine. AfricaRenewal Online. Retrieved from http://www.un.org/africarenewal/magazine/january-2006/traditional-healers-boost-primary-health-care
70. Stanley, B. (2004, February 13). Recognition and Respect for African Traditional Medicine. Canada's International Development Research Centre.
71. Wilkinson, K. (2013, July 31). Do 80% of S. Africans regularly consult traditional healers? The claim is false.
72. Mahmoud, A. H., & El Anany, A. M. (2014). Nutritional and sensory evaluation of a complementary food formulated from rice, faba beans, sweet potato flour, and peanut oil. Food Nutr Bull., 35(4):403-413.
73. Oruamabo, R. S. (2015). Child malnutrition and the Millennium Development Goals: much haste but less speed? Arch Dis Child. 100 Suppl 1:S19-22.
74. Govindji, A. & Dharamshi, S. (2010). Healthy eating, West African style. Nutrition Centre.
75. Schönfeldt, H. C., & Gibson, H. N. (2012). Dietary protein quality and malnutrition in Africa. Br J Nutr. 2012 Aug;108 Suppl 2:S69-76.
76. United Nations Environment Programme (2012). Agriculture and development in Africa.
77. Fran Osseo-Asare, F. (2005). Food Culture in Sub-Saharan Africa, 138-157. Westport, CT: Greenwood Press
78. www.unmillenniumproject.org (n.d.). Fast Facts: The Faces of Poverty.
79. Phillip, A. (2014, August, 5). Why West Africans keep hunting and eating bush meat despite Ebola concerns. The Washington Post.

80. Brashares, J. S., Arcese, P., Sam, M. K., Coppolillo, P. B., Sinclair, A. R. E., & Balmford, A. (2004). Bushmeat Hunting, Wildlife Declines, and Fish Supply in West Africa. Science, 306(5699), 1180-1183.
81. Wolfe, N. D., Daszak, P., Kilpatrick, A. M., & Burke, D. S. (2005). Bushmeat Hunting, Deforestation, and Prediction of Zoonotic Disease, 11(12).
82. Gaayeb, L., Sarr, J. B., Cames, C., Pinçon, C., Hanon, J. B., Ndiath, M. O.,…Hermann, E. (2014). Effects of malnutrition on children's immunity to bacterial antigens in Northern Senegal. Am J Trop Med Hyg., 90(3), 566-573.
83. Manary, M. (2013). Protein source and quality in therapeutic foods affect the immune response and outcome in severe acute malnutrition. Food Nutr Bull., 34(2), 256-258.
84. Thobakgale, C. F., Fadda, L., Lane, K., Toth, I., Pereyra, F., Bazner, S.,… Altfeld M. (2012). Frequent and strong antibody-mediated natural killer cell activation in response to HIV-1 Env in individuals with chronic HIV-1 infection. J Virol., 86(12), 6986-6993.
85. Gong, L., Maiteki-Sebuguzi, C., Rosenthal, P. J., Hubbard, A. E., Drakeley, C. J., Dorsey, G., & Greenhouse, B. (2012). Evidence for both innate and acquired mechanisms of protection from Plasmodium falciparum in children with sickle cell trait. Blood,119(16), 3808-3814.
86. Faurholt-Jepsen, D., Range, N., PrayGod, G., Jeremiah, K., Faurholt-Jepsen, M., Aabye, M. G.,… Friis, H. (2012). The role of diabetes on the clinical manifestations of pulmonary tuberculosis. Trop Med Int Health, 17(7):877-883.
87. United Nations Human Settlements Programme. (2011). Infrastructure for economic development and poverty reduction in Africa. UN-HABITAT.
88. Aker, J. C. & Mbit, I. M. (2010). Mobile Phones and Economic Development in Africa. Journal of Economic Perspectives 24(3), Summer, 207–232.
89. African Development Bank. (2013). Mortality in Africa: The Share of Road Traffic Fatalities
90. United Nations Department of Economic and Social Affairs. (2014). International decade for action "Water for life." Un.org

91. UNICEF and World Health Organization. (2008). A Snapshot of Drinking Water in Africa. A regional perspective based on new data from the WHO/UNICEF Joint Monitoring Programme for Water Supply and Sanitation.
92. The Economist. (2012). The future of healthcare in Africa. The Economist Intelligence Unit.
93. International Labour Organization. (n.d.). Facts on social security in Africa. www.ilo.org
94. United Nations. (2012). The Millennium Development Goals Report 2012. MDG.
95. Sun, L. H., Dennis, B., Bernstein, L. & Achenbach, J. (2014 October 4). Out of control: How the world's health organizations failed to stop the Ebola disaster. The Washington Post.
96. Penney, J. (2014). Update 4-Mali quarantines dozens as second Ebola outbreak spreads in country. Retrieved from http://www.reuters.com/article/2014/11/12/health-ebola-mali-idUSL6N0T22ZX20141112
97. Vora, N. M., Arthur, R. R., Swerdlow, D. L., & Angulo, F. J. (2015, January 24-30). Preparation of at-risk West African countries for Ebola. The Lancet, 385(9965), 329–330.
98. Ayodele, T., Cudjoe, F., Nolutshungu, T. A., & Sunwabe, C. K. (2005). African Perspectives on Aid: Foreign Assistance Will Not Pull Africa Out of Poverty. Economic Development Bulletin No. 2.
99. Akonor, K. (2008). Foreign aid to Africa: A hollow hope? International law and politics, 40(107), 1071-1078.
100. The National Democratic Institute. (n.d.). Transparency and good governance in African extractive industries.
101. Tambo, E. (2014). Non-conventional humanitarian interventions on Ebola outbreak crisis in West Africa: health, ethics and legal implications. Infect Dis Poverty, 3(1):42
102. European Union of Medical Specialists. (1993). Charter on training of medical specialists in the European community.
103. Drazen, J. M., Campion, E. W., Rubin, E. J., Morrissey, S., & Baden, L. R. (2015). Ebola in West Africa at One Year — From Ignorance to Fear to Roadblocks. N Engl J Med., 372, 563-564.
104. Summers, A., Nyenswah, T. G., Montgomery, J. M., Neatherlin, J., Tappero, J. W., T N, M F, M M., & Centers for Disease Control and Prevention (CDC). (2014, December 19). Challenges in responding

to the ebola epidemic -four rural counties, Liberia, August-November 2014. MMWR Morb Mortal Wkly Rep., 63(50), 1202-1204.
105. Hayden, E. C. (2014, December 15). Infectious disease: Ebola's lost ward. A hospital in Sierra Leone has struggled to continue its research amid the worst Ebola outbreak in history. Nature News Feature, 513(7519).
106. World Health Organization. (2014). Field Situation: How to conduct safe and dignified burial of a patient who has died from suspected or confirmed Ebola virus disease.
107. Centers for Disease Prevention and Control. (2015, February 11). Guidance for safe handling of human remains of Ebola patients in U. S. hospitals and mortuaries.
108. Shears, P., & O'Dempsey, T. J. (2015). Ebola virus disease in Africa: epidemiology and nosocomial transmission. J Hosp Infect., pii: S0195-6701(15)00046-8.
109. Osungbade, K. O., & Oni AA. (2014). Outbreaks-of Ebola virus disease in the West African sub-region. Afr J Med Med Sci., 43(2), 87-97.
110. Wilson Center. (2012). Instability in West Africa: Issues and Challenges to Development and International Security. Woodrow Wilson International Center for Scholars.
111. Ikome, F. N. (2012). Africa's International Borders as Potential Sources of Conflict and Future Threats to Peace and Security. Africa Center for Strategic Studies.
112. Minteh, B. & Perry, A. (2013). Terrorism in West Africa -Boko Haram's evolution, strategy and affiliations. Presented at the Mid-West Political Science Association's 71st Annual Conference Palmer House Hotel, Chicago Illinois.
113. Goita, M. (2011). West Africa's growing terrorist threat: Confronting AQIM's sahelian strategy. Africa security brief. A publication of the Africa center for trategic studies.
114. U.S. Department of State. (n.d.). Country Reports on Terrorism 2013: Chapter 2. Country Reports: Africa Overview. www.state.gov
115. Onuoha, F. C. & Ezirim, G. E. (2013). "Terrorism" and Transnational Organised Crime in West Africa. Al Jazeera Centre for Studies.
116. United Nations High Commission on Refugees. (n.d.). Current dynamics of displacement.

117. Hoeffler, A. (2008). Dealing with the consequences of violent conflicts in Africa. Background Paper for the African Development Bank Report 2008.
118. Sabes-Figuera, R., McCrone, P., Bogic, M., Ajdukovic, D., Franciskovic, T., Colombini, N.,...Priebe, S. (2012). Long-term impact of war on healthcare costs: an eight-country study. PLoS ONE 7(1): e29603.
119. Whitty, C. J. M., Farrar, J., Ferguson, N., Edmunds, W. J., Piot, P., Leach, M. & Davies, S. C. (2014, November 6). Infectious disease: Tough choices to reduce Ebola transmission. Nature Comment, 515(7526).
120. The Economist. (2014, October 18). Much worse to come. The Ebola epidemic in west Africa poses a catastrophic threat to the region, and could yet spread further.
121. Eardley, W., Bowley, D., Hunt, P., Round, J., Tarmey, N., & Williams, A. (2015). Education and Ebola: initiating the cascade of emergency healthcare training. J R Army Med Corps., pii: jramc-2014-000394.
122. Chukwuneke, F. N., Ezeonu, C. T., Onyire, B. N., & Ezeonu, P. O. (2012). Culture and biomedical care in Africa: the influence of culture on biomedical care in a traditional African society, Nigeria, West Africa. Niger J Med., 21(3), 331-333.
123. World Health Organization. (n.d.). Cross-border health risks. Trade, foreign policy, diplomacy and health.
124. Suk, J. E., Van Cangh, T., Beauté, J., Bartels, C., Tsolova, S., Pharris, A.,...Semenza, J. C. (2014). The interconnected and cross-border nature of risks posed by infectious diseases. Global Health Action, 7.
125. Alexander, K. A., Sanderson, C. E., Marathe, M., Lewis, B. L., Rivers, C. M., Shaman, J.,...Eubank, S. (2014). What Factors Might Have Led to the Emergence of Ebola in West Africa? PLOS Neglected Tropical Diseases.
126. Koroma, D. (2015). Ebola outbreak in Sierra Leone: Waterloo Adventist Hospital experience (Unpublished).
127. Wonacott, P. (2014, November, 17). Africa's village healers complicate Ebola fight: In Sierra Leone, traditional treatments and death of a woman who resisted outside help fostered outbreak. Retrieved from http://www.wsj.com/articles/africas-village-healers-complicate-ebola-fight-1416268426

128. World Health Organization. (n.d.). Sierra Leone: a traditional healer and a funeral: More than 300 Ebola cases link back to one funeral. Global Alert and Response (GAR)
129. Tchacondo, T., Karou, S. D., Batawila, K., Agban A, Ouro-Bang'na, K., Anani, K. T.,…de Souza C. (2011). Herbal remedies and their adverse effects in Tem tribe traditional medicine in Togo. Afr J Tradit Complement Altern Med., 8(1):45-60.
130. Kollie-Jones, T. (2014). Exploring the power of money, faith-healing, and position in West Africa (Unpublished).
131. Ross, W. (2014, October 20). Ebola crisis: How Nigeria's Dr Adadevoh fought the virus. Retrieved from http://www.bbc.com/news/world-africa-29696011
132. Sieh, R. D. (2014, July 31). Sawyer's Final Hours In Lagos: 'Indiscipline', rage, strange. Retrieved from http://frontpageafricaonline.com/index.php/news/2506-awyer-s-final-hours-in-lagos-indiscipline-rage-strange
133. Fishman, B. M., Bobo, L., Kosub, K., & Womeodu, R. J. (1993). Cultural issues in serving minority populations: emphasis on Mexican Americans and African Americans. Am J Med Sci., 306(3), 160-166.
134. Juckett, G. (2005). Cross-cultural medicine. Am Fam Physician, 1;72(11), 2267-2274.
135. Jerving, S. (2014, September 16). Why Liberians Thought Ebola Was a Government Scam to Attract Western Aid. Retrieved from http://www.thenation.com/article/181618/why-liberians-thought-ebola-was-government-scam-attract-western-aid
136. International Crisis Group. (2014, September 23). Statement on Ebola and Conflict in West Africa. Retrieved from www.crisisgroup.org
137. Rohwerder, B. (2014). Impact and implications of the Ebola crisis. GSDRC Helpdesk Research Report 1177, 1-10.
138. Estrada, C. (2014). Ebola, snakes and witchcraft: Stopping the deadly disease in its tracks in West Africa. Retrieved from www.ifrc.org
139. Hogan, C. (2014, July 18). 'There is no such thing as Ebola.' The Washington Post.
140. Haglage, A. (2014, August 13). Kissing the Corpses in Ebola Country. Retrieved from www.thedailybeast.com

141. Ejizu, C. I. (n.d.). African traditional religions and the promotion of community-living in Africa.
142. Davidson, B. (1969). The African Genius, Boston, P.3
143. Ray, B. (1976). African Religions, Symbol, Ritual and Community. Upper Saddle River, NJ: Prentice-Hall.
144. Eyetsemitan, F. (2002). Suggestions regarding the cross-cultural environment as context for human development and aging in non-Western cultures. Psychological Reports, 90, 823-833.
145. Grundy, T. (2014, September 28). Tradition of kissing, touching corpses may contribute to spread of Ebola, Experts Say. www.huffingtonpost.com
146. Bayntuna, C., Houlihana, C. & Edmundsa, J. (2014). Ebola crisis: beliefs and behaviours warrant urgent attention. Lancet, 384(9952), 1424.
147. Tuomainen, H. (2014). Eating alone or together? Commensality among Ghanaians in London. Anthropology of food [Online], S10. Retrieved from http://aof.revues.org/7718
148. Sobal, J. (2000). Sociability and meals: Facilitation, commensality and interaction. In: MEISELMAN, H. L. (ed.) Dimensions of the meal. The science, culture, business, and art of eating. Gaithesburg: Aspen Publishers, Inc.
149. Konner M. 1981. Evolution of human behavior development. In RH Monroe, R Monroe and JM Whiting (eds): Handbook of cross-cultural development. New York: Garland STPM Press.
150. Whiting, J. (1994). Culture and Human Development: The Selected Papers of John Whiting, Chasdi, E. H. (Ed.), 221-223. NY, NY: Cambridge University Press.
151. Chaplin, K. (n.d.). The Ubuntu spirit in African communities.
152. Duranti, A. (1997). Universal and culture-specific properties of greetings. Journal of Linguistic Anthropology, 7(1), 63-97.
153. Akindele, F. (1990). A sociolinguistic analysis of Yoruba greetings. African Languages and Cultures, 3(1), 1-14.
154. Elladbest.blogspot.com. (2013). Cultures" (The Igbo's, Hausa's, and Yoruba's culture): Interaction, learning, and acknowledgment.
155. Cooper, H. (2014, October 4). Ebola's Cultural Casualty: Hugs in Hands-On Liberia. The New York Times.
156. Gehman, R. J. (2005). African Traditional Religion in Biblical Perspective. Kenya: Autolitho Ltd., 57-80.

157. Tembo, M. S. (n.d.). The Traditional African Family. Retrieved from bridgewater.edu
158. Oosthuizen, G. C. (1988). Interpretation of demonic power in Southern African independent churches, Missiology, XVI(1).
159. Idowu, E. B. (1962). Olodumare: God in Yoruba Belief, 146-150. London: Longman.
160. Gyekye, K. (1997). Tradition and Modernity: Philosophical Reflections on the African Experience, 11-106. NY, NY: Oxford University Press.
161. Zulu, E. M., Konseiga, A., Darteh, E., & Mberu, B. (2006) Migration and urbanization of poverty in sub-Saharan Africa: the case of Nairobi city Kenya [Unpublished]. Presented at the 2006 Annual Meeting of the Population Association of America, Los Angeles, California, March 30 -April 1, 2006.
162. Aaby, P., Bukh, J., Lisse, I. M., & Smits, A. J. (1983). Spacing, crowding, and child mortality in Guinea-Bissau. Lancet, 2(8342), 161.
163. Murove, M. F. (2005). The Incarnation of Max Weber's Protestant Ethic and the Spirit of Capitalism in Post-Colonial Sub-Saharan African Economic Discourse: The Quest for an African Economic Ethic. Mankind Quarterly, 45(4), Summer.
164. Grills, C. T. (2006). Strategies for Psychological Survival & Wellness. African Centered Psychology.
165. Mitman, G. (2014, November, 6). Ebola in a Stew of Fear. N Engl J Med., 371, 1763-1765.
166. Adamo, D. T. (2011).Christianity and the African traditional religion(s): The postcolonial round of engagement. Verbum et Ecclesia 32(1), Art. #285.
167. Alamu, A. G. (n.d.).The place of African ancestors in the age of modernity.
168. Awolalu, J. O. & Dopamu, P. A. (1979). West African Traditional Religion, 247. Ibadan, Oyo State: Onibonje Press and Books Ltd.
169. British Broadcasting Corporation. (2014, August 17). Ebola crisis: Confusion as patients vanish in Liberia. BBC News Africa.
170. The Associated Press. (2014, August 17). Ebola fears rise in Liberia as clinic looted, bloody sheets stolen. Retrieved from www.nydailynews.com

171. Masango, M. J. S. (2005).Cremation a problem to African people. HTS 61(4), 1285-1297.
172. McNeil, D. (2014). Would Cremation Help Stop the Spread of Ebola? United Nations General Assembly. Retrieved from www.nydailynews.com
173. Sobel, M. (1979). Trabelin' On: The Slave Journey to an Afro-Baptist Faith. Greenwood Press.
174. Brooks, C. (2011). Exploring the Material Culture of Death in Enslaved African Cemeteries in Colonial Virginia and South Carolina. African Diaspora Archaeology Newsletter, 14(3).
175. Terry, L. (n.d.). Burying the Peculiar Institution: An analysis of West Tennessee slave culture and religion through cemeteries.
176. Smith, J. (2009). Hidden and Sacred: African-American cemeteries in Eastern North Carolina.
177. Dockins, P. (2014, August 2). WHO: Traditional burials hamper Ebola fight. www.voanews.com
178. Lomax, S. (2014, September 14). Handling Dead: Ebola burial teams stigmatized in Liberia. Retrieved from http://www.frontpageafricaonline.com
179. Actionaid. (2014). The Ebola Effect: Death, Stigma and Economic Hardship. Retrieved from www.actionaidusa.org
180. Mickleburgh, S., Waylen, K., & Racey, P. (2009). Bats as bushmeat: a global reivew. Oryx, 43 (2009), pp. 217–234
181. Kamins, A. O. Restifa, O., Ntiamoa-Baiduc, Y., Suu-Ired, R., Haymana, D. T. S., Cunninghamb, A. A.,…Rowcliffeb, J. M. (2011). Characteristics and risk perceptions of Ghanaians potentially exposed to bat-borne zoonoses through bushmeat. Biological Conservation, 144(12), 3000–3008
182. Mbete, R. A., Banga-mboko, H., Racey, P., Mfoukou, I., Doucet, J., Hornick, J., & Leroy, P. (2011). Household bushmeat consumption in Brazzaville, the Republic of the Congo. Tropical Conservation Science, 4, 187–202.
183. Worldbank.org. (n.d.). Poverty. Retrieved from http://data.worldbank.org/topic/poverty
184. McCracken, G. F. (1992). Bats in magic, potions, and medicinal preparations. Fall, Vol. 10, No. 3.

185. Kasso, M. & Balakrishnan, M. (2013). Ecological and economic importance of bats (Order Chiroptera). International Scholarly Research Notices Biodiversity, 2013(187415), 9 pages.
186. Schleuning, W. D. (2000). Vampire bat plasminogen activator DSPA-alpha-1 (desmoteplase): a thrombolytic drug optimized by natural selection. Pathophysiology of Haemostasis and Thrombosis, 31, 118–122.
187. Publishers, S., Parker, J., Mills, A., & Stanton, J. (2003). Mythology: Myths, legends and fantasies, 277-321. Global Book Publishing Pty Ltd.
188. Idowu, E. B. (1973). African traditional religion: A definition, 12-15. Maryknoll, NY:Orbis Books.
189. van Wagtendonk, A. (2014, August 18). Liberian mob attacks Ebola clinic; dozens of patients missing. PBS Newshour. Retrieved from www.pbs.org
190. Fantz, A. (2014, August 18). Ebola facility in Liberia attacked; patients flee. Retrieved from www.cnn.com
191. Zinnah, S. K. (2007). Corruption engulfs Sea and Airports in Liberia. The perspective. Retrieved from liberiaitech.com
192. Charlton, C. (2014, October 14). Bribery breaks out in battle against Ebola: Liberian victims' families paying corrupt retrieval teams to keep bodies so they can give them traditional burials. Retrieved from www.dailymail.co.uk
193. Farge, E. (2015). Sierra Leone to prosecute fraudulent Ebola "ghostworkers". Retrived from http://news.yahoo.com/sierra-leone-prosecute-fraudulent-ebola-ghostworkers-112831761--business.html
194. Lau, R., Wang A., Chong-Kit, A., Ralevski, F., & Boggild, A. K. (2015). Evaluation of Ebola virus inactivation procedures for plasmodium falciparum malaria diagnostics. J Clin Microbiol. 2015 Jan 28. pii: JCM.00165-15.
195. Bociaga-Jasik, M., Piatek, A., & Garlicki, A. (2014). Ebola virus disease -pathogenesis, clinical presentation and management. Folia Med Cracov., 54(3), 49-55.
196. Drazen, J. M., Campion, E. W., Rubin, E. J., Morrissey, S., & Baden, L. R. (2015). Ebola in West Africa at One Year — From Ignorance to Fear to Roadblocks. N Engl J Med 2015; 372:563-564.
197. McKay, B. & Hinshaw, D. (2014, October 2). Lack of qualified staff hurts Ebola fight in Africa. Wall Street Journal, http://

online.wsj.com/articles/lack-of-qualified-staff-hurts-ebola-fight-in-africa-1412293011 (accessed Oct 6, 2014).
198. Irikefe, V., Vaidyanathan, G., Nordling, L., Twahirwa, A., Nakkazi, E. & Monastersky, R. (2011). Nature, 474, 556-559.
199. Comte, M. (2014, October 18). Lab half a world away at center of West Africa Ebola fight. Retrieved from news.yahoo.com
200. Salaam-Blyther, T. (2014, October 29). U.S. and International Health Responses to the Ebola Outbreak in West Africa. Congressional Research Service, 7-5700, www.crs.gov R43697.
201. United Nations Development Programme (2014). Ebola Crisis in West Africa. Retrieved from http://www.undp.org/content/undp/en/home/ourwork/our-projects-and-initiatives/ebola-response-in-west-africa.html
202. Regan, H. (2015, February 16). Schools in Liberia Reopen After a Six-Month Closure Due to Ebola. Retrieved from www.time.com
203. Isaac I Bogoch, I. I., Creatore, M. I., Cetron, M. S., Brownstein, J. S., Pesik, N., Miniota, J.,...Khan, K. (2014). Assessment of the potential for international dissemination of Ebola virus via commercial air travel during the 2014 West African outbreak. The Lancet, 385(9962), 29–35.
204. Carod-Artal, F. J. (2015). Illness due the Ebola virus: epidemiology and clinical manifestations within the context of an international public health emergency. Rev Neurol., 60(6), 267-277.
205. Vigliotti, M. (2014). Lambton College Ebola screening complete. Retrieved from www.thesarniajournal.ca
206. Alabi, C. (2014). Nigeria: Kaduna schools complain over Ebola screening equipment. Daily Trust.
207. Neporent, L. (2014, September 30). Nigerian Ebola hoax results in two deaths. Retrieved from abcnews.go.com
208. Ezeobi, C. (2014, August 9). Nigeria: 'We Pranked on Salt-Water Therapy' As FG Debunks Claims. This Day.
209. Gonda, D. D., Meltzer, H. S., Crawford, J. R., Hilfiker, M. L., Shellington, D. K., Peterson, B. M., Levy, M. L. (2013). Complications associated with prolonged hypertonic saline therapy in children with elevated intracranial pressure. Pediatr Crit Care Med., 14(6), 610-620.

210. Frisoli, T. M., Schmieder, R. E., Grodzicki, T., Messerli, F. H. (2012). Salt and hypertension: is salt dietary reduction worth the effort? Am J Med., 125(5):433-439.
211. Wagner, M. (2014, August 16). Phony Ebola cures spread online; 2 Nigerians die from drinking salt water to ward off virus, UN says. Retrieved from www.nydailynews.com
212. World Health Organization. (2014). Ebola: Experimental therapies and rumoured remedies. Retrieved from http://www.who.int/mediacentre/news/ebola/15-august-2014/en/
213. Fauci, A. & Kresge, K. J. (2014). Battling Ebola: the virus and the fear. IAVI Rep., 8(4), 11-13.
214. Millard, W. B. (2015). Gallows humor, fearmongering continue to spread. Ann Emerg Med., 65(2), 21A-22A.
215. Judah, S. (2014, August 6). The Ebola 'cure' that offers false hope. BBC Trending. www.bbc.com
216. Channels Television. (2014, August 19). Ebola: Bitter kola stops replication of virus, not a cure. Retrieved from http://www.channelstv.com/2014/08/19/ebola-bitter-kola-stops-replication-virus-cure/
217. Fung, I. C., Tse, Z. T., Cheung, C. N., Miu, A. S., Fu, K. W. (2014). Ebola and the social media. Lancet, 384(9961), 2207.
218. Yoder-Wise PS. (2014). Blame free-"Bah, humbug!" the need for responsible media about Ebola. J Contin Educ Nurs., 45(11), 475-476.
219. Sim, F. & Mackie, P. (2014). The rising tide of Ebola. Public Health, 128(9), 769-770.
220. Salmon, S., McLaws, M. L., & Fisher, D. (2015). Community-based care of Ebola virus disease in West Africa. Lancet Infect Dis., 15(2), 151-152.
221. Ippolito, G., Puro, V., & Piselli, P. (2015). Ebola in West Africa: who pays for what in the outbreak? New Microbiol., 38(1), 1-3.
222. Rodriguez-Morales, A. J., Castañeda-Hernández, D. M., McGregor, A. (2015). What makes people talk about Ebola on social media? A retrospective analysis of Twitter use. Travel Med Infect Dis., 13(1), 100-101.
223. United Nations. (2015). Ebola: World Bank reports economic impact in worst-hit countries to exceed $500 million in 2014. Retrieved from http://www.un.org/apps/news/story.asp?NewsID=49490#.VNRNNtE5DIU

224. Food and Agriculture Organization. (2015). Ebola Outbreak West Africa: FAO Response Programme (October 2014 – September 2015) -Updated version January 2015. www.fao.org
225. United Nations Population Fund. (2015). Ebola Virus Disease Outbreak in West Africa -January 2015 update. www.unfpa.org
226. Mulrine, A. (2015, February 11). With Ebola cases down dramatically, US military ends mission in West Africa. Retrieved from http://www.csmonitor.com/USA/Military/2015/0211/With-Ebola-cases-down-dramatically-US-military-ends-mission-in-West-Africa-video
227. Lushniak, B. D. (2015). Update on the u.s. Public health response to the ebola outbreak. Public Health Rep., Mar-Apr,130(2), 118-120.
228. Madariaga, M. G. (2015). Ebola virus disease: a perspective for the United States. Am J Med., pii: S0002-9343(15)00167-9.
229. US Department of State. (n.d.). Office of the Historian. Milestones: 1830–1860: Founding of Liberia, 1847. Retrieved from https://history.state.gov/milestones/1830-1860/liberia
230. UK. (n.d.). UK action plan to defeat ebola in Sierra Leone: Background paper: An international call for assistance. Retrieved from https://www.gov.uk/government/uploads/system/uploads/attachment_data/file/35 7703/UK_action_plan_to_defeat_Ebola_in_Sierra_Leone_-_background_paper.pdf
231. Sierra-Leone.org. (1996-2015). Welcome to the Sierra Leone web. Retrieved from http://www.sierra-leone.org/facts.html
232. Smith-Spark, L. & Akhoun, L. (2014, November 28). France's President Francois Hollande visits Ebola-stricken Guinea. Retrieved from http://www.cnn.com/2014/11/28/world/africa/guinea-france-hollande-ebola/
233. British Broadcasting Corporation. (n.d.). Guinea profile. Retrieved from http://www.bbc.com/news/world-africa-13443183
234. Economic Community of West Africa States. (n.d.). Synergy of efforts: key to containing ebola epidemic in the ECOWAS region. Retrieved from http://www.wahooas.org/spip.php?article711&lang=en
235. African Union. (n.d.). Fact sheet: African union response to the Ebola epidemic in West Africa. Retrieved from http://pages.au.int/ebola/documents/fact-sheet-african-union-response-ebola-epidemic-west-africa
236. Cidi.org. (n.d.). Non-Governmental Organizations Responding to the Ebola Crisis. www.cidi.org

237. Georgetown Journal of International Affairs (2014). NGOs, Ebola, and the future of civil actors in international politics: five minutes with Sam Worthington. www.journal.georgetown.edu
238. Arie, S. (2014). MSF: how a humanitarian charity found itself leading the world's response to Ebola. BMJ., 349, g7737.
239. Vogel, L. (2014). Call for Ebola medics falls on deaf ears: MSF. CMAJ., 186(18), E669.
240. World Health Organization. (2014, July-December).WHO strategic action plan for Ebola outbreak response. www.who.int
241. Tomori, O. (2014). Ebola in an unprepared Africa. BMJ, 349, g5597.
242. White, R. A., MacDonald, E., de Blasio, B. F., Nygård, K., Vold, L., & Røttingen, J. A. (2015. Projected treatment capacity needs in Sierra Leone. PLoS Curr., pii: ecurrents. outbreaks.3c3477556808e44cf41d2511b21dc29f.
243. Takahashi, S., Metcalf, C. J., Ferrari, M. J., Moss, W. J., Truelove, S. A., Tatem, A. J.,…Lessler J. (2015). Reduced vaccination and the risk of measles and other childhood infections post-Ebola. Science, 347(6227), 1240-1242.
244. Gettleman, J. (2014, December 30). Ebola Ravages Economies in West Africa. www.nytimes.com
245. Columbus, F. H. (Ed.). 2001). Politics and Economics of Africa (Vol. 1), pp. 18-33. Huntington, NY: Nova Science Publishers, Inc.
255. Bolkan, H. A., Bash-Taqi, D. A., Samai, M., Gerdin, M., & von Schreeb, J. (2014). Ebola and Indirect Effects on Health Service Function in Sierra Leone. PLoS Current Outbreaks.
256. World Health Organization. (2014). Sierra Leone: Helping the Ebola survivors turn the page. Retrieved from http://www.who.int/features/2014/post-ebola-syndrome/en/
257. United Nations International Children's Emergency Fund (2015). Ebola response. www.unicef.org
258. Hessou, C. (2015). Ebola survivors facing stigma, unemployment, exclusion. www.unfpa.org
259. Elbagir, N. & Brumfield, B. (2014, October 20). Ebola makes stigmatized, abandoned orphans. Retrieved from http://www.cnn.com/2014/10/20/world/africa/ebola-liberia-orphans/index.html
260. Gettleman, J. (2014, December, 13). An Ebola orphan's plea in Africa: 'Do you want me?' Retrieved from http://www.nytimes.

com/2014/12/14/world/africa/an-ebola-orphans-plea-in-africa-do-you-want-me.html?_r=0
261. Proshareng.com. (2014, August 16). Making Economic Sense of the Ebola Scare -How it affects each sector.
262. Abdullah, A. A. (2011). Trends and Challenges of Traditional Medicine in Africa. Afr J Tradit Complement Altern Med., 8(5 Suppl), 115–123.
263. Sack, K., Fink, S., Belluck, P. & Nossiter, A. (2014, December 29). How Ebola roared back. www.nytimes.com
264. UN News Center. (n.d.). Powerful effects of Ebola outbreak felt outside worst-affected countries. www.ebolaresponse.un.org
265. Mylott, E. (2009). Urban-Rural Connections: A Review of the Literature. www.ir.library.oregonstate.edu
266. Meissner, O. (2004). The traditional healer as part of the primary health care team? S Afr Med J., 94(11), 901-902.
267. United Nations Development Programme (2014). Assessing the socio-economic impacts of Ebola Virus Disease in Guinea, Liberia and Sierra Leone: The road to recovery. Retrieved from www.africa.undp.org/.../EVD%
268. Bausch, D. G. & Schwarz, L. (2014). Outbreak of ebola virus disease in Guinea: where ecology meets economy. PLoS Negl Trop Dis., 8(7), e3056.
269. WHO Ebola Response Team. (2014). Ebola virus disease in West Africa — the first 9 months of the epidemic and forward projections. N Engl J Med., 371, 1481-1495.
270. Mahesh, R. (2015, February 5). Post-Ebola Syndrome: Survivors Report Memory Loss, Chest Pain, Mental Illness, Eye Problems. www.ibtimes.co.in
271. World Bank. (2015). The Socio-Economic Impacts of Ebola in Liberia. www.worldbank.org
272. United Nations Development Programme. (2015). West African economies feeling ripple effects of Ebola, says UN. www.undp.org
273. Garrett, L. (2014, October 10). Five myths about Ebola. The Washington Post.
274. The Editorial Board. (2014, August 6). Ebola myths range from dumb to deadly: Our view. www.usatoday.com
275. Giraldi, G. & Marsella, L. T. (2015). Ebola Virus Disease Outbreak: What's going on. Ann Ig., 27(1), 82-6.

276. Fhogartaigh CN, Aarons E. (2015). Viral haemorrhagic fever. Clin Med.,15(1), 61-66.
277. Sharfstein, J. M. (2015). On fear, distrust, and Ebola. JAMA, 313(8), 784.
278. Mundasad, S. (2014, September 22). Ebola virus: Busting the myths. www.bbc.com
279. Karamouzian, M. & Hategekimana, C. (2014). Ebola treatment and prevention are not the only battles: understanding Ebola-related fear and stigma. Int J Health Policy Manag., 4(1), 55-56.
280. Lee-Kwan, S. H., DeLuca, N., Adams, M., Dalling, M., Drevlow, E., Gassama, G.,…Centers for Disease Control and Prevention (CDC). (2014). Support services for survivors of ebola virus disease -Sierra Leone, 2014. MMWR Morb Mortal Wkly Rep., 63(50), 1205-1206.
281. Farge, E. & Giahyue, J. H. (2015, February 5). Free from Ebola, survivors complain of new syndrome. www.reuters.com
282. Royal African Society. (2014). The West African Ebola Outbreak: Gaps in governance and accountability. www.royalafricansociety.org
283. Wiwanitkit, V., Tambo, E., Ugwu, E. C., Ngogang, J. Y., & Zhou, X. N. (2015). Are surveillance response systems enough to effectively combat and contain the Ebola outbreak? Infect Dis Poverty, 4(1), 7.
284. Chabot-Couture, G., Seaman, V. Y., Wenger, J., Moonen, B., & Magill, A. (2015). Advancing digital methods in the fight against communicable diseases. Int Health, 7(2), 79-81.
285. World Health Organization. (2014). The outbreak of Ebola virus disease in Senegal is over. Retrieved from http://www.who.int/mediacentre/news/ebola/17-october-2014/en/
286. Weintraub, K. (2014). From Senegal and Nigeria, 4 Lessons on how to stop Ebola. www.nationalgeographic.com
287. World Health Organization. (2014). Nigeria is now free of Ebola virus transmission. Retrieved from http://www.who.int/mediacentre/news/ebola/20-october-2014/en/
288. Summers, A., Nyenswah, T. G., Montgomery, J. M., Neatherlin, J., Tappero, J. W. (2014). Challenges in Responding to the Ebola Epidemic — Four Rural Counties, Liberia, August–November 2014. Morbidity and Mortality Weekly Report, 63(50), 1202-1204.
289. Zavis, A. (2014, October 22). Ebola-free: How did Nigeria and Senegal do it? www.latimes.com

290. Mason, J. P. (1989). The role of urbanization in national development: Bridging the rural-urban divide. U.S. Agency for International Development. A.I.D. Program evaluation discussion paper no. 27.
291. Hove, M., Ngwerume, E. T., & Muchemwa, C. (2013). The Urban Crisis in Sub-Saharan Africa: A Threat to Human Security and Sustainable Development. Stability: International Journal of Security and Development, 2(1), 7.
292. Misra, T. (2014). Does Ebola Spread Faster in Cities? www.citylab.com
293. Schnirring, L. (2014). CDC assessment cites rural gaps in Liberia's battle with Ebola. Center for Infectious Disease Research and Policy. www.cidrap.umn.edu
294. Asuzu, M. C., Onajole, A. T., Disu, Y. (2015). Public health at all levels in the recent Nigerian Ebola viral infection epidemic: lessons for community, public and international health action and policy. J Public Health Policy
295. Grigg, C., Waziri, N. E., Olayinka, A. T., Vertefeuille, J. F. (2015). Use of group quarantine in ebola control -Nigeria, 2014. MMWR Morb Mortal Wkly Rep, 64(5), 124.
296. Kunii, O., Kita, E., & Shibuya, K. (2001). Epidemics and related cultural factors for Ebola hemorrhagic fever in Gabon. Nihon Koshu Eisei Zasshi, 48(10), 853-859.
297. Beaubien, J. (2014). Firestone did what governments have not: Stopped Ebola in its tracks. www.npr.org
298. French, H. W. (2013). How Africa's new urban centers are shifting its old colonial boundaries. www.theatlantic.com
299. Boone, C. (2003). Decentralization as political strategy in West Africa. Comparative Political Studies, 36(4), 355-380.
300. Ribot, J. C. (2002). African decentralization local actors, powers and accountability. UNRISD Programme on Democracy, Governance and Human Rights Paper Number 8.
301. World Health Organization. (2014, November 10). Mali case, Ebola imported from Guinea. Retrieved from http://www.who.int/mediacentre/news/ebola/10-november-2014-mali/en/
302. World Health Organization. (2014, October 24). Mali confirms its first case of Ebola. Retrieved from http://www.who.int/mediacentre/news/ebola/24-october-2014/en/

303. World Health Organization. (2014, November 20). Mali: Details of the additional cases of Ebola virus disease. Retrieved from http://www.who.int/mediacentre/news/ebola/20-november-2014-mali/en/
304. World Health Organization. (2014, November). WHO Director-General visits Mali to bolster UN support to the Ebola outbreak. Retrieved from http://www.who.int/features/2014/dg-mali-visit/en/
305. Westcott, L. (2015). Mali Declared Ebola-Free By WHO. www.newsweek.com
306. World Health Organization. (2014, October, 23). Summary report of a WHO High-level meeting on Ebola vaccines access and financing. Retrieved from http://www.who.int/mediacentre/news/ebola/23-october-2014/en/
307. CBC.ca. (2014, August 12). Canada offers experimental Ebola vaccine VSV-EBOV to West Africa: Canada has about 1,500 doses of the vaccine and will donate as many as 1,000 to WHO. Retrieved from http://www.cbc.ca/news/health/canada-offers-experimental-ebola-vaccine-vsv-ebov-to-west-africa-1.2734681
308. ClinicalTrials.gov. (2015). Safety, tolerability, and immunogenicity of the Ebola chimpanzee adenovirus vector vaccine (cAd3-EBO), VRC-EBOADC069-00-VP, in healthy adults. Retrieved from https://www.clinicaltrials.gov/ct2/show/NCT02231866?term=NCT02231866&rank =1
309. Grover, N. (2014, February 12). Novavax starts Ebola vaccine trial in humans. Retrieved from http://www.reuters.com/article/2015/02/12/us-health-ebola-novavax-idUSKBN0LG1NX20150212
310. National Institutes of Health. (2014, November 28). NIAID/GSK experimental Ebola vaccine appears safe, prompts immune response. Results from NIH Phase 1 clinical trial support accelerated development of candidate vaccine. Retrieved from http://www.nih.gov/news/health/nov2014/niaid-28.htm
311. Parry, L. (2014, November 14). First nasal spray Ebola vaccine found "offer long-term protection against deadly virus." Retrieved from http://www.dailymail.co.uk/health/article-2820202/First-nasal-spray-Ebola-vaccine-offer-long-term-protection-against-deadly-virus.html
312. Pharmiweb.com. (2015). Vaxart Completes Financing to Fund Expanding Development Portfolio Vaxart. Retrieved from http://

www.pharmiweb.com/pressreleases/pressrel.asp?ROW_ID=106188#. VOr M7tE5DIV

313. Philippidis, A. (2014, September 4). GEN News Highlights: J&J/Bavarian Nordic, NewLink Plan Trials for Ebola Vaccines. Retrieved from http://www.genengnews.com/gen-news-highlights/j-j-bavarian-nordic-newlink-plan-trials-for-ebola-vaccines/81250305/

314. WHO (2015g, January 21): Essential medicines and health products: Ebola vaccines, therapies, and diagnostics: Questions and Answers. Retrieved from http://www.who.int/medicines/emp_ebola_q_as/en/

315. Hayden, E. C. (2014 August, 28). Ebola virus mutating rapidly as it spreads: Outbreak likely originated with a single animal-to-human transmission. Nature News. Retrieved from http://www.nature.com/news/ebola-virus-mutating-rapidly-as-it-spreads-1.15777

316. Mazumdar, T. (2015, January 29). Ebola outbreak: Virus mutating, scientists warn. Retrieved from http://www.bbc.com/news/health-31019097

317. Bellan, S. E, Pulliam, J. R., Dushoff, J., & Meyers, L. A. (2014). Ebola control: effect of asymptomatic infection and acquired immunity. Lancet, 384(9953), 1499-1500.

318. Hodge, J. G. Jr., Gostin, L. O., Hanfling, D., & Hick, J. L.(2015). Law, medicine, and public health preparedness: the case of Ebola. Public Health Rep., 130(2):167-170.

319. Gulland, A. (2014). UK built Ebola treatment centre opens in Sierra Leone. BMJ, 349, g6704.

320. Hill, C. E., Burd, E. M., Kraft, C. S., Ryan, E. L., Duncan, A., Winkler, A. M.,…Parslow TG. (2014). Laboratory test support for ebola patients within a high-containment facility. Lab Med., Summer, 45(3), e109-11.

321. Wendo, C. (2003). African countries to cooperate on epidemic control. Experts hope that sharing expertise and resources will help control disease outbreaks in the region. Lancet, 362(9379), 222.

322. Piot, P., Muyembe, J. J., & Edmunds, W. J. (2015). Ebola in West Africa: from disease outbreak to humanitarian crisis. Lancet Infect Dis., 14(11), 1034-1035.

323. Caplan, A. L. (2015). Morality in a time of Ebola. Lancet, pii: S0140-6736(14)61653-61656.

324. Resnik, D. B. (2011). What is Ethics in Research and Why is it Important? Retrieved from http://www.niehs.nih.gov/research/resources/bioethics/whatis/
325. Kissinger, D. (2014). Scandal-driven research ethics (Unpublished).
326. McWhirter, R. E. (2012). The history of bioethics: implications for current debates in health research. Perspect Biol Med., 55(3), 329-338.
327. Gallin, J. I., & Ognibene, F. P. (Eds.). (2012). *Principles and practice of clinical research* (3rd ed.), pp. 19-42. Waltham, MA: Academic Press.
328. Nelson, C. R. (2012). In remembrance there is prevention: A brief review of four historical failures to protect human subjects. Journal of Research Administration, 43(1).
329. Centers for Disease Control and Prevention. (2013). U.S. Public Health Service Syphilis Study at Tuskegee: Presidential apology: The White house. Retrieved from http://www.cdc.gov/tuskegee/clintonp.htm
330. U.S. Department of Health and Human Services. (1979). The Belmont Report. Retrieved from http://www.hhs.gov/ohrp/humansubjects/guidance/belmont.html
331. Joffe, S. (2015). Ethical testing of experimental ebola treatments--reply. JAMA, 313(4), 422.
332. World Health Organization. (2000). World Health Organization Assesses the World's Health Systems. World Health Report. Retrieved from http://www.who.int/whr/2000/media_centre/press_release/en/
333. Lindblad, R., El Fiky, A., & Zajdowicz, T. (2014). Ebola in the United States. J Allergy Clin Immunol., pii: S0091-6749(14)01792-01798.
334. Afolabi, M. O., Okebe, J. U., McGrath, N., Larson, H. J., Bojang, K., & Chandramohan, D. (2014). Informed consent comprehension in African research settings. Trop Med Int Health, 19(6), 625-642.
335. Purcaru D, Preda A, Popa D, Moga MA, Rogozea L. (2014). Informed consent: how much awareness is there? PLoS One, 9(10), e110139.
336. Herper, M. (2013 August 11). The cost of creating a new drug now $5 billion, pushing big pharma to change. Forbes' Pharma & Healthcare. Retrieved from http://www.forbes.com/sites/matthewherper/2013/08/11/how-the-staggering-cost-of-inventing-new-drugs-is-shaping-the-future-of-medicine/

337. Surowiecki, J. (2014, August 25). Ebolanomics. The New Yorker. Retrieved from http://www.newyorker.com/magazine/2014/08/25/ebolanomics
338. Millman, J. (2014, August 13). Why the drug industry hasn't come up with an Ebola cure. The Washington Post. Retrieved from http://www.washingtonpost.com/blogs/wonkblog/wp/2014/08/13/why-the-drug-industry-hasnt-come-up-with-an-ebola-cure/
339. Hofmarcher, T. & Borg, S. (2015). Cost-effectiveness analysis of ferric carboxymaltose in iron-deficient patients with chronic heart failure in Sweden. J Med Econ., 1-20.
340. World Health Organization. (2014). Ethical considerations for use of unregistered interventions for Ebola virus disease: Report of an advisory panel to WHO. Retrieved from http://www.who.int/csr/resources/publications/ebola/ethical-considerations/en/
341. Food and Drug Administration. (2014). Investigational new drug (IND) application. Retrieved from http://www.fda.gov/drugs/developmentapprovalprocess/howdrugsaredevelopeda ndapproved/approvalapplications/investigationalnewdrugindapplication/default.htm
342. Centers for Disease Control and Prevention. (2015). 2014 Ebola Outbreak in West Africa -Case Counts. Retrieved from http://www.cdc.gov/vhf/ebola/outbreaks/2014-west-africa/case-counts.html
343. Von Drehle, D. & Baker, A. (2014, December 22-29). The ones who answered the call. Time, 184(24-25), 70-6, 78, 80-2 passim.
344. Satalkar, P., Elger, B. E., & Shaw, D. M. (2015). Prioritising healthcare workers for Ebola treatment: Treating those at greatest risk to confer greatest benefit. Dev World Bioeth.
345. Dynes, M. M., Miller, L., Sam, T., Vandi, M. A., Tomczyk, B, & Centers for Disease Control and Prevention (CDC). (2015, January 2). Perceptions of the risk for Ebola and health facility use among health workers and pregnant and lactating women--Kenema District, Sierra Leone, September 2014. MMWR Morb Mortal Wkly Rep., 63(51), 1226-1227.
346. Strauss, S. (2014). Ebola research fueled by bioterrorism threat. CMAJ, 186(16), 1206.
347. Kosal, M. E. (2014). A new role for public health in bioterrorism deterrence. Front Public Health, 2, 278.
348. Rosoff, P. M. (2015). In defense of (some) altered standards of care for ebola infections in developed countries. HEC Forum, 27(1), 1-9.

349. Fox, M. (2014, August 21). What Cured Ebola Patients Kent Brantly and Nancy Writebol? Retrieved from http://www.nbcnews.com/storyline/ebola-virus-outbreak/what-cured-ebola-patients-kent-brantly-nancy-writebol-n186131
350. Food and Drug Administration. (2015). Expanded Access: Information for patients. Retrieved from http://www.fda.gov/ForPatients/Other/ExpandedAccess/ucm20041768.htm
351. Rahbari, M. & Rahbari, N. N. (2011). Compassionate use of medicinal products in Europe: current status and perspectives. Bulletin of the World Health Organization, 89 (3), 161-240. Retrieved from http://www.who.int/bulletin/volumes/89/3/10-085712/en/#
352. Gaffney, A. (2013). New FDA draft guidance aims to clarify compassionate use process. Retrieved from http://www.raps.org/regulatoryDetail.aspx?id=8489#sthash.sBjvThFr.dpuf
353. Krech, R. & Kieny, M. P. (2014). The 2014 Ebola outbreak: ethical use of unregistered interventions. Bull World Health Organ., 92(9), 622.
354. Dawson, A. J. (2015). Ebola: What it tells us about medical ethics. J Med Ethics, 41(1), 107-110.
355. Gillon, R. (2015). Defending the four principles approach as a good basis for good medical practice and therefore for good medical ethics. J Med Ethics, 41(1), 111-116.
356. Nijhawan, L. P., Janodia, M. D., Muddukrishna, B. S., Bhat, K. M., Bairy, K. L., Udupa, N., & Musmade, P. B. (2013). Informed consent: Issues and challenges. J Adv Pharm Technol Res., 4(3), 134-140.
357. Grady, C. (2015). Enduring and emerging challenges of informed consent. N Engl J Med, 372(9), 855-862.
358. Różyńska, J. (2015). On the Alleged Right to Participate in High-Risk Research. Bioethics.
359. Neuman, G., Shavit, I., Matsui, D., & Koren, G. (2015). Ethics of research in pediatric emergency medicine. Paediatr Drugs, 17(1), 69-76.
360. DeWitt, D. E, Ward, S. A., Prabhu, S., & Warton B. (2009). Patient privacy versus protecting the patient and the health system from harm: a case study. Med J Aust., (4), 213-216.
361. Zhai, H., Zhong, W., & Wu, Y. (2015). Research, evidence, and ethics: new technology or grey medicine. Ann Transl Med, 3(2), 15.
362. Péron, J., Roy, P., Ding, K., Parulekar, W. R., Roche, L., & Buyse, M. (2015). Assessing the benefit-risk of new treatments using generalised

pairwise comparisons: the case of erlotinib in pancreatic cancer. Br J Cancer.
363. Sabo, S., de Zapien, J., Teufel-Shone, N., Rosales, C., Bergsma, L, Taren, D. (2015). Service learning: a vehicle for building health equity and eliminating health disparities. Am J Public Health, 105 Suppl 1, S38-43.
364. Torabi-Parizi, P., Davey, R. T. Jr, Suffredini, A. F., Chertow, D. S. (2015). Ethical and practical considerations in providing critical care to patients with Ebola virus disease. Chest.
365. Lucchini, R. G. & London, L. (2014). Global occupational health: current challenges and the need for urgent action. Ann Glob Health, 80(4), 251-256.
366. Maurice, J. (2014). WHO meeting chooses untried interventions to defeat Ebola. The Lancet, 384(9948), e45–e46,
367. Fauci, A. S. (2014). Ebola—underscoring the global disparities in health care resources. N Engl J Med, 371 (2014), pp. 1084–1086
368. Markel, H. (2014). Ebola fever and global health responsibilities. Milbank Q., 92(4), 633-639.
369. McMurry, E. (2014, November 4). WHO Director criticizes 'profit-driven' pharma industry for ignoring Ebola vaccine. www.mediaite.com
370. Food and Drug Administration. (2013). Orphan Drug Act. Retrieved from http://www.fda.gov/regulatoryinformation/legislation/federalfooddrugandcosmetic actfdcact/significantamendmentstothefdcact/orphandrugact/default.htm
371. Bailey, J. (2014). Monkey-based research on human disease: The implications of genetic differences. Alternatives to Laboratory Animals (ATLA), 42(5), 287-317.
372. Perkel, J. M. (2012). Animal-free toxicology: Sometimes, in vitro is better. Science: Life Science Technologies. Retrieved from http://www.sciencemag.org/site/products/lst_20120302.xhtml
373. Greek, R., Shanks, N., & Rice, M. J. (2011). The history and implications of testing Thalidomide on animals. The Journal of Philosophy, Science & Law, 11
374. Physicians Committee for Responsible Medicine. (2005). Vioxx tragedy spotlights failure of animal research. Retrieved from ttp://www.pcrm.org/media/online/mar2005/vioxx-tragedy-spotlights-failure-of-animal

375. Akhtar, A. (2012). Animals and public health: Why treating animals better is critical to human welfare. Basingstoke, UK: MacMillan
376. Pippin, J. J. (2014). The Failing Animal Research Paradigm for Human Disease. Independent Science News.
377. DeGraba, T. J., & Pettigrew, L. C. (2000). Why do neuro-protective drugs work in animals but not humans? Neurol Clin., 18(2), 475-493.
378. Hayden, E. C. (2014, March 26). Misleading mouse studies waste medical resources. Retrospective of more than 100 failed drugs show many should have never made it to clinical trials. Nature News. Retrieved from http://www.nature.com/news/misleading-mouse-studies-waste-medical-resources-1.14938
379. Sena, E. S., van der Worp, H. B., Bath, P. M. W., Howells, D. W., & Macleod, M. R. (2010). Publication bias in reports of animal stroke studies leads to major overstatement of efficacy. PLoS Biology. Retrieved from http://journals.plos.org/plosbiology/article?id=10.1371/journal.pbio.1000344
380. California Biomedical Research Association. (n.d.). Why are animals necessary in biomedical research? www.ca-biomed.org
381. Johnson, J. A., & Bootman, J. L. (1995). Drug-related morbidity and mortality. A cost-of-illness model. Arch Intern Med, 155(18), 1949–1956.
382. Leape, L. L., Brennan, T. A., Laird, N., Lawthers, A. G., Localio, A. R., Barnes, B. A.,...Hiatt, H. (1991). The nature of adverse events in hospitalized patients. Results of the Harvard Medical Practice Study II. N Engl J Med., 324(6), 377– 384.
383. Classen, D. C., Pestotnik, S. L., Evans, R. S., Lloyd, J. F., Burke, J. P. (1997). Adverse drug events in hospitalized patients. Excess length of stay, extra costs, and attributable mortality. JAMA, 277(4), 301–306.
384. Shapiro, H. T. (2001). Ethical and policy issues in research involving human participants. Volume II Commissioned Papers and Staff Analysis, Bethesda, Maryland August 2001, National Bioethics Advisory Commission.
385. Goldie, P., Döring, S. & Cowie, R. (2011). The ethical distinctiveness of emotion-oriented technology: Four long-term issues. Emotion-Oriented Systems
Cognitive Technologies, pp. 725-733
386. Pruett, T. L., Tibell, A., Alabdulkareem, A., Bhandari, M., Cronin, D. C., Dew, M. A.,... Francis L. Delmonico, F. L. (2006). The ethics

statement of the vancouver forum on the live lung, liver, pancreas, and intestine donor. Transplantation, 81(10), 1386-1387.
387. Bialas, W. & Fritze, L. (2014). Nazi Ideology and Ethics, pp. 193-306. London, UK: Cambridge Scholars Publishing.
388. O'Mathúna, D. P. (2006). Human dignity in the Nazi era: Implications for contemporary bioethics. BMC Medical Ethics, 7:2.
389. Annas, G. J. & Grodin, M. A. (Eds.). (1995). Book Review: The Nazi doctors and the Nuremberg Code. J. Pharmacy & Law. LexisNexis.
390. Kortepeter, M. G., Smith, P. W., Hewlett, A. & Cieslak, T. J. (2015). Caring for patients with Ebola: A Challenge in any care facility. Ann Intern Med., 162(1), 68-69.
391. Rid, A. & Emanuel, E. J. (2014). Ethical considerations of experimental interventions in the Ebola outbreak. The Lancet, 384(9957), 1896–1899.
392. Kim, W. O. (2012). Institutional review board (IRB) and ethical issues in clinical research. Korean J Anesthesiol., 62(1), 3–12.
393. Karp, B. I. (2012). Purpose and function of IRBS: Successes and challenges. CNS IRB, NIH.
394. Council for International Organizations of Medical Sciences. (2002). International ethical guidelines for biomedical research involving human subjects. Bull Med Ethics, 182, 17-23.
395. Fosså, S. D. & Skovlund, E. (2000). Interim analyses in clinical trials: Why do we plan them? JCO., 18(24), 4007-4008.
396. Sica, D. A. (2002).Premature termination of clinical trials--lessons learned. J Clin Hypertens (Greenwich), 4(3), 219-225. Review.
397. Fadare, J. O. & Porteri, C. (2010). Informed consent in human subject research: A comparison of current international and Nigerian guidelines. J Empir Res Hum Res Ethics, 5(1), 67-73.
398. Montenegro, S. A. & Monreal, A. M. E. (2008). The informed consent in international clinical trials including developing countries. Cuad Bioet., 19(65), 67-79.
399. Kass NE, Maman S, Atkinson J. (2005). Motivations, understanding, and voluntariness in international randomized trials. IRB, 27(6), 1-8.
400. Bhutta, Z. A. (2004). Beyond informed consent. Bull World Health Organ., 82(10), 771-777. Review.
401. Ansmann, E. B., Hecht, A., Henn, D. K., Leptien, S., & Stelzer, H. G. (2013). The future of monitoring in clinical research -a holistic approach: linking risk-based monitoring with quality management principles. Ger Med Sci., 11, Doc04.

402. Marsolo K. (2012). Approaches to facilitate institutional review board approval of multicenter research studies. Med Care, 50 Suppl:S77-81.
403. Levchuk, J. W. (1991). Good manufacturing practices and clinical supplies. J Parenter Sci Technol., 45(3), 152-155.
404. de Maar, E. W., Chaudhury, R. R., Kofi, E. J. M., Granata, F., & Walker, A. N. (1983). Management of clinical trials in developing countries. J Int Med Res.,11(1), 1-5.
405. Prokscha, S. (2012). Practical guide to clinical data management (3rd Ed.), pp. 103-111. Boca Raton, FL: CRC Press.
406. Yue, L. Q., Lu, N., & Xu, Y. (2014). Designing premarket observational comparative studies using existing data as controls: challenges and opportunities. J Biopharm Stat., 24(5), 994-1010.
407. Gupta, A. (2013). Fraud and misconduct in clinical research: A concern. Perspect Clin Res., 4(2), 144–147.
408. Turner, J. R. (2007). New Drug Development: Design, methodology, and analysis, pp. 165-183. Hoboken, NJ: John Wiley & Sons, Inc.
409. Fhogartaigh, C. N. & Aarons, E. (2015). Viral haemorrhagic fever. Clin Med., 15(1), 61-66.
410. Marzi, A. & Feldmann, H. (2014). Ebola virus vaccines: An overview of current approaches. Expert Rev Vaccines, 13(4), 521-531.
411. Centers for Disease Control and Prevention (2014). Detailed Emergency Medical Services (EMS) checklist for Ebola preparedness.
412. Wong, G., Qiu, X., Olinger, G. G., & Kobinger, G. P. (2014). Post-exposure therapy of filovirus infections. Trends Microbiol., 22(8), 456-463.
413. Presidential Commission for the Study of Bioethical Issues. (2015). Ethics and Ebola public health planning and response.
414. World Health Organization (2015 January). WHO Ebola R&D Effort – vaccines, therapies, diagnostics (Update). Retrieved from http://www.who.int/medicines/ebola-treatment/ebola_r_d_effort/en/
415. Touitou, Y., Portaluppi, F., Smolensky, M. H, & Rensing, L. (2004). Ethical principles and standards for the conduct of human and animal biological rhythm research. Chronobiology International, 21(1), 161-170.
416. Ng, Rick. Drugs: From Discovery to Approval, 2nd ed., 19-51, 208-396. Hoboken: John Wiley & Sons, Inc., 2009.

417. DeRenzo, Evan G. and Moss, Joel. Writing Clinical Research Protocols: Ethical Considerations, 1-26. Burlington: Elsevier Academic Press, 2006.
418. Michael, N. (2002). Greek medicine: The Hippocratic Oath. National Library of Medicine.
419. World Health Organization. (2014). Sierra Leone: Increasing community engagement for Ebola on-air. Retrieved from http://www.who.int/features/2015/radio-messages-ebola/en/
420. World Health Organization. (2014). Government of Senegal boosts Ebola awareness through SMS campaign. Retrieved from http://www.who.int/features/2014/senegal-ebola-sms/en/
421. World Health Organization. (2014). Infection prevention and control guidance summary: Ebola guidance package. Retrieved from http://www.who.int/csr/resources/publications/ebola/evd-guidance-summary/en/
422. Nielsen, C. F., Kidd, S., Sillah, A. R. M., Davis, E., Mermin, J. & Kilmarx, P. H. (2015). Improving burial practices and cemetery management during an Ebola virus disease epidemic -Sierra Leone, 2014. CDC Morbidity and Mortality Weekly Report (MMWR), 64(01), 20-27.
423. Centers for Disease Control and Prevention. (2015). Infection Prevention and Control Recommendations for Hospitalized Patients Under Investigation (PUIs) for Ebola Virus Disease (EVD) in U.S. Hospitals (Updated). Retrieved from http://www.cdc.gov/vhf/ebola/healthcare-us/hospitals/infection-control.html
424. Public Health Agency of Canada. (2014). Public Health Management of Cases and Contacts of Human Illness Associated with Ebola Virus Disease (EVD). www.publichealth.gc.ca
425. World Health Organization. (2014). Contact tracing during an outbreak of Ebola virus disease: Disease surveillance and response programme area disease prevention and control cluster. WHO Regional Office for Africa.
426. World Health Organization. (2014). Laboratory diagnosis of Ebola virus disease. WHO/EVD/GUIDANCE/LAB/14.1
427. Lewnard, J. A., Mbah, M. L. N., Alfaro-Murillo, J. A., Altice, F. L., Bawo, L., Nyenswah, T. G., Galvani, A. P. (2014). Dynamics and control of Ebola virus transmission in Montserrado, Liberia:

a mathematical modelling analysis. Lancet Infectious Diseases, 14(12), 1189.
428. World Health Organization Country Office for Thailand. (2014). Ebola virus disease. Retrieved from http://www.searo.who.int/thailand/factsheets/fs0034/en/
429. Centers for Disease Control and Prevention. (2015). Questions and answers about Ebola, pets, and other animals. Retrieved from http://www.cdc.gov/vhf/ebola/transmission/qas-pets.html
430. Roland, T. S. (Ebola Virus Disease (EVD) Outbreak in West Africa: The Nigerian Experience. Rolex Global Consult.
431. The European Commission. (n.d.).Questions and answers on foot and mouth disease. Retrieved from http://ec.europa.eu/food/animal/diseases/controlmeasures/qa_fmd_en.print.htm
432. Centers for Disease Control and Prevention. (2015). Questions and Answers on Ebola. Retrieved from http://www.cdc.gov/vhf/ebola/outbreaks/2014-west-africa/qa.html
433. American Evaluation Association. (2011). Public Statement on Cultural Competence in Evaluation. Fairhaven, MA: Author. Retrieved from www.eval.org
434. Lewens, T. (2013). Stanford Encyclopedia of Philosophy: Cultural evolution. Retrieved from http://plato.stanford.edu/entries/evolution-cultural/
435. Taflinger, R. F. (1996). Human cultural evolution. Retrieved from http://public.wsu.edu/~taflinge/culture1.html
436. Jonathan, S. (2001). The Search for Modern China. NY, NY: W.W. Norton & Co.
437. The Editors of Encyclopædia Britannica. (2015). Industrial Revolution. Retrieved from http://www.britannica.com/EBchecked/topic/287086/Industrial-Revolution
438. DeWoskin, K. J. (2015). China: The Cultural Revolution, 1966–76. Retrieved from http://www.britannica.com/EBchecked/topic/111803/China/71852/The-Cultural-Revolution-1966-76
439. Shackel, P. A. (1996). Culture change and the new technology: An archaeology of the early American industrial era, pp. 1-16. NY, NY: Plenum Press.
440. Wilson, D. (1997). Traditional systems of communication in modern African development an analytical viewpoint. Africa Media Review, 1(2), 87-104.

441. Lazuta, J. (2013, January 28). Report: Mobile Phones Transform Lives in Africa. Retrieved from http://www.voanews.com/content/woldbank-reports-says-mobile-phones-transform-lives-in-developing-africa/1592270.html
442. Norton, M. R. & Addy, M. (1989). Chewing sticks versus toothbrushes in West Africa. A pilot study. Clin Prev Dent., 11(3), 11-13.
443. Hooda, A., Rathee, M., & Singh, J. (2009). Chewing sticks in the era of toothbrush: A Review. The Internet Journal of Family Practice, 9(2).
444. Akinyemi, A. (2011). African oral tradition then and now: A culture in transition. Centrepoint Journal (Humanities Edition), 14(1).
445. Moody, A. (2001). Electronic media in Africa. Final paper. Media Technologies and Society. Fall 2001.
446. Blog.culturalecology.info. (2013). Cultural ecology: Cultural entropy – Maintaining order.
447. Louppe, D., Oteng-Amoako, A. A., & Brink, M. (Eds.). (2008). Plant resources of tropical Africa: Timbers, pp. 560-580. Wageningen, Netherlands: PROTA Foundation.
448. Garrity, D., Dixon, J., & Boffa, J. (2012). Understanding African farming systems: Science and policy implications. www.aciar.gov.au
449. World Bank. (2013). Protecting West African fisheries: Improving access for locals and regional management. www.worldbank.org
450. Leavitt M. (2014). Learning the lessons of Ebola as events continue to unfold. Mod Healthc., 44(43), 26.
451. Klein, E. J. (2008).Learning, unlearning, and relearning: Lessons from one school's approach to creating and sustaining learning communities. Teacher Education Quarterly, Winter 2008.
452. World Health Organization. (2014). New WHO safe and dignified burial protocol -key to reducing Ebola transmission. Retrieved from http://www.who.int/mediacentre/news/notes/2014/ebola-burial-protocol/en/
453. Sachdeva, V. (n.d.).Good documentation and quality management principles. www.who.int
454. World Health Organization. (n.d.). Communicable disease prevention, control and eradication. Retrieved from http://www.afro.who.int/en/ethiopia/country-programmes/communicable-diseases.html
455. Sandle, T. (2014). Good documentation practices. Retrieved from http://www.ivtnetwork.com/article/good-documentation-practices

456. Avruch, K. (1998). Culture and conflict resolution. United States Institute of Peace, Washigton, DC.
457. World Health Organization, Regional Office of Africa. (2015, March 20).Empowering communities to conduct safe burial practices. Retrieved from http://www.afro.who.int/en/liberia/press-materials/item/7487-empowering-communities-to-conduct-safe-burial-practices.html
458. Pless, N. & Maak, T. (2004). Building an inclusive diversity culture: Principles, processes and practice. Journal of Business Ethics, 54(2), pp. 129-147.
459. Inglehart, R. (1990). Culture shift in advanced industrial society, 26-31. Princeton, NJ: Princeton University Press.
460. Saltman, R. B., Bankauskaite, V., & Vrangbaek, K. (2007). Decentralization in health care, NY, NY: Open University Press.
461. Hewlett, B. S. & Amola, R. P. (2003). Cultural contexts of Ebola in Northern Uganda. Emerg Infect Dis., 9(10), 1242–1248.
462. Schnirring, L. (2014, December 19). UN head tours Ebola region, warns against let-up. CIDRAP News. Retrieved from http://www.cidrap.umn.edu/news-perspective/2014/12/un-head-tours-ebola-region-warns-against-let
463. World Health Organization. (2014). Frequently asked questions on Ebola virus disease. Global Alert and Response (GAR). Retrieved from http://www.who.int/csr/disease/ebola/faq-ebola/en/
464. Centers for Disease Control and Prevention. (2014, November 20). Ebola. National Center for Emerging and Zoonotic Infectious Disease.
465. Wodon, Q. (2007). Growth and Poverty Reduction: Case Studies from West Africa. Washington, DC: World Bank.
466. Shamoo, A. E. (2015, January 19). Ebola – Yes to isolation, quarantine, and travel restrictions (Part II). Retrieved from http://www.bioethics.net/2015/01/ebola-yes-to-isolation-quarantine-and-travel-restrictions-part-ii/
467. Urban, A. (2015, March 16). Liberia honors cremated Ebola victims. Global Communities. Retrieved from http://www.globalcommunities.org/node/38066
468. Fink, S. & Belluck, P. (2015, March 22). One Year Later, Ebola outbreak offers lessons for next epidemic. www.nytimes.com

469. Axelrod, R. (1997). The dissemination of culture a model with local convergence and global polarization. Journal of Conflict Resolution, 41(2), 203-226.
470. Musisi, S. & Musisi, N. (n.d.). The legacies of colonialism in African medicine. www.who.int/global_health
471. Pinkoane, M. G., Greeff, M., & Koen, M. P. (2012). A model for the incorporation of the traditional healers into the national health care delivery system of South Africa. Afr J Tradit Complement Altern Med., 9(3 Suppl), 12-18.
472. World Health Organization. (2012). WHO traditional medicine strategy: 2014-2023. www.who.int
473. Waitzkin, H., Iriart, C., Estrada, A., & Lamadrid, S. (2001). Social medicine then and now: Lessons from Latin America. Am J Public Health, 91(10), 1592–1601.
474. WebMD. (2005-2015).Complementary and alternative medicine (CAM) Overview. Retrieved from http://www.webmd.com/balance/what-is-alternative-medicine
475. Chitindingu, E., George, G., & Gow, J. (2014). A review of the integration of traditional, complementary and alternative medicine into the curriculum of South African medical schools. BMC Medical Education, 14, 40.
476. Guan, A. & Chen, C. A. (n.d.). Integrating traditional practices into allopathic medicine. The Journal of Global Health.
477. Ben-Arye, E., Scharf, M., & Frenkel, M. (2007). How should complementary practitioners and physicians communicate? A cross-sectional study from Israel. Journal of the American Board of Family Medicine, 6, 565-571.
478. Occupational Safety & Health Administration. (n.d.). Control and prevention. Retrieved from https://www.osha.gov/SLTC/ebola/control_prevention.html
479. Engler, R. L., Covell, J. W., Friedman, P. J., Kitcher, P. S., & Peters, R. M. (1987). Misrepresentation and responsibility in medical research. New England Journal of Medicine 317:1383-1389.
480. Lachman, V. D., Murray, J. S., Iseminger, K. & Kathryn M. Ganske, K. M. (2012). Doing the right thing: Pathways to moral courage. www.americannursetoday.com

481. Bostick, N. A., Mark A. Levine, M. A., & Sade, R. M. (2008). Ethical obligations of physicians participating in public health quarantine and isolation measures. Public Health Rep., 123(1), 3–8.
482. Chin, J. (Ed.). (2000). Control of communicable diseases manual (17th ed.) (Selected excerpts). Washington: American Public Health Association.
483. Gostin, L. O. (2014).Ebola: Towards an international health systems fund. The Lancet, September 2014.
484. Government of the United Kingdom. (2014, December 17). Global Health Systems Remain "Dangerously Inadequate" For Dealing With Health Emergencies Like Ebola, Says Committee. Retrieved from http://reliefweb.int/report/sierra-leone/global-health-systems-remain-dangerously-inadequate-dealing-health-emergencies
485. World Health Organization. (2015 February). Keeping communities safe from contaminated waste. Retrieved from http://www.who.int/csr/en/
486. Laplante, P. A. (2004).First, do no harm: A Hippocratic Oath for software developers. What's wrong with taking our profession a little more seriously?, Development, 2(4).
487. Brubaker, R. (2004). In the name of the nation: Reflections on nationalism and patriotism. Citizenship studies, 8(2),115-127.
488. WAHOOAS.org. (2009). About WAHO: History and Missions. Retrieved from http://www.wahooas.org/spip.php?page=rubriqueS&id_rubrique=24&lang=en
489. Economic Community of West Africa States. (n.d.). ECOWAS community development programme (CDP): Concept Note. www.cdp-pcd.ecowas.int
490. Asante S.K.B., (2012). Challenges and opportunities of regional integration for developing economies. Issues in African Regional Integration -2012. Center for Regional Integration in Africa (CRIA). Ghana Institute of Management and Public Administration (GIMPA).
491. Lodge, J. (1994). "Transparency and Democratic Legitimacy." Journal of Common Market Studies, 32: 45-69
492. Olubomehin D. and Kawonishe D. (2008). The African Union and the Challenges of Regional Integration in Africa. African Renewal, African Renaissance': New Perspectives on Africa's Pastand Africa's Present. The African Studies Association of Australia and the Pacific

(AFSAAP) Annual Conference 26-28 November 2004, University of Western Australia.
493. World Bulletin. (2014, December 15). ECOWAS leaders discuss Ebola, terror challenges. Retrieved from http://www.worldbulletin.net/haber/150841/ecowas-leaders-discuss-ebola-terror-challenges
494. African Studies Centre (n.d.). Privatization in Africa. Retrieved from http://www.ascleiden.nl/content/webdossiers/privatization-africa
495. Mbonye, A. K., Wamala, J. F., Nanyunja, M., Opio, A., Makumbi, I., & Aceng, J. R. (2014). Ebola viral hemorrhagic disease outbreak in West Africa-Lessons from Uganda. Afr Health Sci., 14(3), 495–501.
496. UNICEF. (2014, August 12). Fact Sheet: Generation 2030 Africa Report. Retrieved from www.unicef.org/esaro/FINALFactSheetGen 2030Africa.pdf
497. Fleshman, M. (2009). Laying Africa's roads to prosperity. Retrieved from http://www.un.org/africarenewal/magazine/january-2009/laying-africa%E2%80%99s-roads-prosperity
498. Thewaterproject.org. (n.d.).Water scarcity & the importance of water: Learn about access to water and the global water shortage. Retrieved from http://thewaterproject.org/water_scarcity
499. Martin, R. (2015, January 25). Mistrust, anger holds guinea back from fighting Ebola. www.npr.org
500. Triplecrisis.com. (2012, February 27). Rich presidents of poor nations: An African story of oil and capital flight. Retrieved from http://triplecrisis.com/rich-presidents-of-poor-nations/
501. Akinbobola, T. O. & Saibu, M. O. O. (2004). Income inequality, unemployment, and poverty in Nigeria: a vector autoregressive approach. The Journal of Policy Reform, 7(3), 175-183.
502. The Economist. (2012, March 31). African democracy: A glass half-full. Retrieved from http://www.economist.com/node/21551494
503. Bossert, T. (1998). Analyzing the decentralization of health systems in developing countries: decision space, innovation and performance. Soc Sci Med., 47(10), 1513-1527.
504. Smith, B. C. (1997). The decentralization of health care in developing countries: organizational options. Public Administration and Development, 17, 399-412.
505. World Health Organization. (n.d.).First Antigen Rapid Test for Ebola through Emergency Assessment and Eligible for Procurement. Essential medicines and health products. Retrieved from http://

www.who.int/medicines/ebola-treatment/1st_antigen_RT_Ebola/en/

506. World Health Organization. (2008). Patient safety workshop: Learning from error. WHO/IER/PSP/2008.09
507. Imaworldhealth.org. (2015, February 26). Stopping Ebola in its tracks: Maximizing a health system approach for an improved epidemic response: Recommendations from IMA's Experiences Containing Ebola Outbreaks in the DRC.
508. Waterman, S. H., Escobedo, M., Wilson, T., Edelson, P. J., Bethel, J. W., & Fishbein, D. B. (2009). A new paradigm for quarantine and public health activities at land borders: Opportunities and challenges. Public Health Rep., 124(2), 203–211.
509. Thelancet.com. (2015, February 10). Ebola in West Africa: learning the lessons. World Report.
510. Shetty, P. (2010). Integrating modern and traditional medicine: Facts and figures. Retrieved from http://www.scidev.net/global/disease/feature/integrating-modern-and-traditional-medicine-facts-and-figures.html
511. Komesaroff P, Kerridge I. (2014). Ebola, ethics, and the question of culture. J Bioeth Inq., 11(4), 413-414.

List of Contributors

Chief Oyetade Akintubuwa (Olukoyi), Renowned Historian and Head, *Alaghoro* of Ugbo Kingdom, Ilaje Local Government Area, Ondo State, Nigeria, West Africa.

Felix I. Ikuomola, PhD Candidate in Clinical Research Program, John A. Burns School of Medicine, University of Hawaii, Honolulu, Hawaii, USA and Graduate Research Assistant, University of Hawaii Cancer Center, Honolulu, Hawaii, USA. And also pursues MSc in Surgical Sciences at the Royal College of Surgeons of Edinburgh and University of Edinburgh, UK. Already obtained an MS in Clinical Research. Had a surgery residency at JFK Medical Center, Monrovia, Liberia. A recipient of NIH Diversity Supplement 2014 award.

Wendy A. Ikuomola, Nursery Nurse, Complementary and Alternative Medicine Therapist, and Medical Missionary, UK.

Trinida A. Kollie-Jones, Family Nurse Practitioner Program, Widener University, PA and Medical Missionary, USA.

David Koroma, Medical Director, Waterloo Hospital, Freetown, Sierra Leone.

Olumide Oluwarotimi, Medical doctor, State Specialist Hospital, Okitipupa, Ondo State and Heritage Alpha Intercontinental Hospital, Ugbo, Ondo State.

Walter C. Thompson, Retired, Surgeon, Family Physician, Author, and Medical Missionary, USA.

Index

A

Accountability, 19, 20, 29, 33, 82, 114
Adverse event, 83
    severe, 80, 84
Africa
    east, xxv, 3, 29, 31, 46, 49, 57
    west, xxv, 3, 5, 6, 8, 13-25
African Traditionalist, 15, 41
    west, 15
Animal
animal-animal, 6
    testing, 6
Assent, 75
Assistance, 20, 23, 33, 42, 47, 129

B

Bat, 6
    eater, 25
    food, 39
    fruit, 6
    taxonomy, 6
Beneficence, 76
Bewitching, 32
Bioethics, 70-85
Bioterrorism, 47, 74, 81
Bitter kola nut, 45, 56, 96
Brain drain, 22
Bribery, 20, 23, 33, 41, 114, 122
Burial, 15, 86, 87
    cemetery, 38, 39
    ground, 38, 39
    Place, 16
    Rites, 15
    Rituals, 33
Bush meat, 6, 25, 33, 37
    Eater, 37

C

CDC, 86, 93, 120
Centrifugal outbreak, 59, 60, 67
Centripetal outbreak, 53, 59, 60, 67
Chlorine, 86, 113
Communication, 27, 28, 59, 68, 108,127
Community, 113
    dialogue, 113, 127, 128
    engagement, 86, 113, 127
Compassionate use, 75
Conclusion, 131-133
Confidentiality, 76
Consent, 71, 72, 75, 76, 82
    informed, 71, 72, 75, 76, 82
Contact tracing, 48, 57, 59-62, 86, 131
    good, 68
    poor, 68, 117
Containment, 59, 60, 74, 77, 87, 90, 131
Corpse, 15, 33, 34, 36, 38
    washing, 33, 34, 115
    preservation, 34
    holding and wailing, 34
Corruption, 19, 20, 23, 33, 41, 67, 114
Cremation, 38, 39, 87, 115
Culture
    evolution, 62, 106, 112, 115

practices, 14, 15, 33, 88, 112
resolution, 63, 106
revolution, 106, 109, 115, 132
traditional, 37, 39, 41, 118
tribes, 13, 14, 21
Cycle, 78
   vicious, 78, 125, 129
   virtuous, 78

D

Decentralization, 124
Diagnosis, 11
   differential, 12, 42
   wrong, 42
Dignity, 36, 71, 76, 81, 84, 115
Double set up, 84

E

Eating custom, 35
Ebola
   epidemiology, 5, 62
   classification, 5
   comparative, 8
   distribution, 8, 50
   complications, 12, 35, 56, 75
   disease burden, 7
   fatality, 1, 8, 29, 74
   fraud, 42, 119
   free, 100, 133
   hemorrhagic fever, 1, 5, 12, 22
   historical account, 1
   incubation period, 1, 43, 54, 61
   investigations, 10-12, 42
   message, 30, 44
   morbidity, 1, 7, 67
   mortality, 1, 7, 8, 17

mutation, 66
myth, 55, 56, 94
outbreak, 1, 3, 5-10, 22
pathogenesis, 10
prognosis, 12, 68, 131
related memories, 88-100
responder, 117, 122
schematic diagram, 11
screening, 44, 60, 69, 95
strains, 8
   Bundibugyo, 1, 2, 5, 8
   Reston, 1, 2, 5, 8
   Sudan, 1, 2, 5, 8
   tai forest, 3, 5, 8
   zaire, 1, 2, 5, 8
surveillance, 47, 48, 57-59, 68
test kits, 124, 125
timeline, 1
transmission, 6, 33-35, 38
   animal-animal, 6
   animal-human, 6
   human-human, 7
treatment, 11, 12, 29
vaccines, 12, 46, 62-63, 70
virus, 1-3, 6-12
Economy, 9, 22, 51, 53, 55
   reduced, 53
Education, 17, 18, 31, 53
   adult literacy, 17, 53, 59
Efficacy, 12, 79
Elijah, 15
Elisha, 15
Empathy, 38, 113, 129
Ethics, 70
   acceptability, 73, 80-81, 84
   application, 71, 72, 77, 81,
   dilemma, 70
   fundamental principles, 71

historical account, 70
  permissible, 75
  principles, 71
  rationale, 72, 77
  soundness, 76, 80-81
Expectatio, 71, 129
Evolution, 62, 106, 112
  culture, 106, 112

F

Faith healer, 113, 117, 118, 126
FDA, 70, 73, 76, 81
Female genital mutilation, 15
Filoviridae, 1, 5

G

Greeting, 36, 93
Guidelines, 59, 87
  animal, 87
  health workers/care givers, 86
  laboratory, 87
  public, 86
  travel warnings, 87
Guinea, 3, 6, 8, 13, 17, 22, 23, 26

H

Hand washing, 34, 35, 86, 90
Health, 9
  care, 9, 24, 43, 48, 53
  center, 23, 26, 42, 43
    insufficient, 23
    malfunctioning, 23
  disparity, 60, 78
  infrastructures, 22, 51, 83, 101
  insurance, 23
  low GDP, 23, 69
  workers, 23, 29-31, 33, 44
Hygiene, 34
  lack, 34, 60,

I

Infection, 1, 11, 60, 86
Infectious disease, 29, 47, 57, 72, 84
Isolation, 29, 37, 38, 41

J

Job, 9, 17
  loss, 9, 54
  urban, 9, 23
Justice, 72, 77
  distributive, 77
  social, 77

K

Kiss, 36, 115
  corpse, 36
  cheek, 36

L

Liberia, 8-10, 13, 19, 22, 23, 26, 48
  storylines, 90-95
Look-listen-learn, 128

M

Magic, 18, 40, 109
Magnanimous norm, 37
Mali, 8, 13, 17, 26, 28, 30, 49, 50
Media, 27, 46, 58-60

Medico-cultural, 131
    disease, 131
    junction, 131
Miracle-healer, 32
MSF, 49

N

Nepotism, 21
Never again, 131
NGO, 49, 60, 69
Nigeria, 8, 10, 13, 18, 19, 22, 23, 99
Nutrition, 24, 50, 55, 67, 72
    unbalanced, 24

O

Orphan drug, 79
Orphans, 52, 90, 132
Overcrowding, 33, 37

P

Patient, 9-11, 22, 23
    index, 3, 32, 58
Personal protective equipment, 29, 48
Pharmacodynamics, 79
Pharmacokinetics, 79
Physician-patient ratio, 22, 51, 52, 68
Post-Ebola syndrome, 52, 56, 57, 75
Poverty, 17, 19, 21, 30, 31
Pragmatism, 60, 83, 84
Pre-clinical, 62, 72, 73, 76
Privacy, 76
Professional responsibility, 119
    5Ps, 119
    patriotism, 120
    peer, 119
    personal, 119
    policy, 120
    public, 120
Prognostic factor, 67, 68
    ebola, 67, 68
    general ebola eradication, 67, 68
    outbreak-type, 67, 68
Proverb, 20

Q

Quarantine, 28, 29, 43, 47, 54, 60

R

Reciprocity, 77, 85
References, 137-175
Religion, 18, 40, 132
    african traditional, 18, 40, 41
    christianity, 18, 132
    islam, 18
    syncretism, 18
Repressive policy, 21
Resolution, 62, 72, 106, 112, 113, 115
    culture, 106, 112, 113, 115
Respect, 15, 71
    basic approach, 126
    person, 72
Revolution, 106
    culture, 106, 109, 112, 115

S

Safety, 12, 64, 76, 78-83
Salt, 44, 45, 56, 95
Sanitation, 26, 86, 93
Senegal, 8, 10, 11, 17, 26, 28, 50, 57
Sharing, 35, 37

bed, 35
deceased personal belongings 41
food, 37
Shrines, 18
Sierra Leone, 8, 9, 13, 17, 19, 22, 23, 48
ebola, 48
storylines, 88-90
Social, 13, 19, 23
amenities, 26, 60, 68, 102
conflict, 19
discrimination, 39, 90
security system, 28
stigmatization, 52, 56, 69, 93
usefulness, 77, 85
war, 19, 23, 67
Storylines, 88-105
Strategy, 130

T

Tax evasion, 21
Terrorism, 74
Togetherness, 16, 35-37, 128
Traditional, 15, 18, 24
healer, 24, 31, 32, 67
healer incorporation program 118
integration, medical program, 118
medicinal practitioner, 118
Transparency, 19, 29, 33

U

Umpteenth, 128
UN, 47
Understanding, 127
Unemployment, 17, 37
Unregistered, 70
interventions, 70

treatment, 70
vaccine, 46, 62, 74

V

Virucidal, 6, 7
Virus, 1, 6-8
ebola, 1

W

WAHO, 48
West Africa, 3,
ecowas, 13, 16,32, 48
ethnic languages, 14
geography, 13
health organization
ifa divination, 14
mission, 13
people, 13
policy, 13
politics, 13
populations, 13
schematic map, 14
total area, 13
WHO, 3, 56-58, 61-63, 100

Y

Yellow fever, 5
Youth, 17
unemployment, 17, 37, 41, 90

Z

Zaire, 1, 3, 5, 7, 50
Zoonosis, 6

Epilogue

Dr. Felix Ikuomola in his book provides clear insight into the social and cultural factors unique to West Africa that had an impact on the Ebola epidemic, including the impact of years of war in the region resulting in destruction and lack of basic infrastructure, and the cultural funerary rituals. This include the cleaning and preparation of the bodies, and the tradition to touch the bodies of the deceased by friends and relatives at the funerals, leading to further contamination of others in the community. In addition, it gives a very comprehensive overview of the economic, medical, epidemiological and other important aspects of this epidemic. The book also provides insights on prevention strategies to control and avoid future epidemics of this deadly disease in Africa and worldwide. This is a great book for anyone who wants to learn about Ebola and the many complex factors that played a role in this epidemic.

Beatriz L. Rodriguez, MD, MPH, PhD
Professor of Geriatric Medicine and
Complementary and Alternative Medicine,
John A. Burns School of Medicine,
University of Hawaii,
Honolulu, HI, USA

Made in the USA
Lexington, KY
07 November 2015